Mike Franklin was educated at ̲ ̲ ̲ ̲ ̲
University of California at B ̲ ̲ ̲ ̲
publishing company at the age of 25 and later ̲ ̲ ̲
California where he worked as a literary agent. He returned to
England four years ago and has since commissioned and edited
many books on health. He has also worked closely with two
doctors specializing in environmental medicine and has his own
practice treating patients with ME.

Jane Sullivan (née Crowther) is an experienced medical and
health writer. She is deputy science editor of the weekly
newspapers *Doctor* and *Hospital Doctor*. She is a regular health
and general feature writer for newspapers and women's magazines, was deputy editor of *The Best of Health* magazine and has
worked widely in medical and science publishing. She has a
degree in botany and psychology from Reading University.

This book is not intended to replace the services of a doctor. Any application of the recommendations set forth in the following chapters is at the reader's discretion.

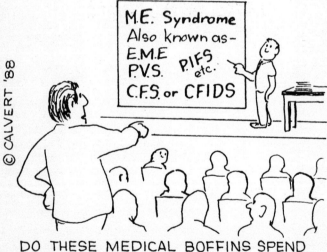

M.E.
WHAT IS IT?
HAVE YOU GOT IT?
HOW TO GET BETTER

MIKE FRANKLIN
AND
JANE SULLIVAN

CENTURY
LONDON SYDNEY AUCKLAND JOHANNESBURG

Copyright © Mike Franklin and Jane Sullivan 1989

All rights reserved

First published in Great Britain in 1989
by Century Hutchinson Ltd
Brookmount House, 62–65 Chandos Place,
Covent Garden, London WC2N 4NW

Century Hutchinson Australia (Pty) Ltd
89–91 Albion Street, Surry Hills
New South Wales 2010, Australia

Century Hutchinson New Zealand Ltd
PO Box 40–086, 32–34 View Road, Glenfield,
Auckland 10, New Zealand

Century Hutchinson South Africa (Pty) Ltd,
PO Box 337, Bergvlei, 2012 South Africa

Typeset by Deltatype Ltd , Ellesmere Port

Printed and bound by The Guernsey Press Ltd,
Guernsey, Channel Islands

British Library Cataloguing in Publication Data

Franklin, Mike
    M. E.
    1. Man. Myalgic encephalomyelitis
    I. Title II. Sullivan, Jane
    616.8'3

ISBN 0 7126 2966 1

Table of Contents

'Each patient carries his own doctor inside him. They come to us not knowing that truth. We are at our best when we give the doctor who resides within each patient a chance to go to work.'

Dr Albert Schweitzer

Acknowledgements

The chapters in this book on allergies and candida albicans and indeed any references to the part played by allergies in the illness myalgic encephalomyelitis would not have been possible without Doctors Mumby, Monro, Kingsley and Mansfield – pioneers in looking at illness from a new point of view.

I should also like to thank especially the two Madeleines, Christine Catley, Angela Watkins and Richard Grant. My grateful thanks also to all those many sufferers who allowed me to interview them and to two doctors whose books have been an invaluable source of reference: Dr Melvin Ramsay, *Post Viral Syndrome: The Saga of Royal Free Disease* and Dr Darrel Ho-Yen, *Better Recovery from Viral Illnesses*.

MF

I would like to thank my sister Ruth Crowther for helping with the manuscript, my boss Dr John DuBois, who gave up his holiday to let me have the time off work and my husband Bill who did the cooking and put up with all my gripes during the writing of this book.

JS

1 Angela's Story

Angela Hawkins was 43 when she contracted ME in 1986. Her husband died of a heart attack two years before, and she has two teenage children with whom she has a close and loving relationship. She had worked as a nurse for many years and considered herself exceptionally fit in that she played tennis four or five times a week – often twice a day. She played anyone, and if there was snow on the ground she would just get out there and sweep the court so that she could play just the same. She had, she says, more energy than most people she knew.

She has always kept a diary, and these are some of her entries from 24 May 1986. If some of the entries seem remarkably lucid for someone ill it should be borne in mind that one of the hallmarks of ME is that the symptoms fluctuate from one day to the next, not to say one hour to the next.

My illness started at the end of May 1986. I had felt really tired for five or six days, and then the next day, when I was playing tennis, I felt very disorientated, had palpitations while on the court and then actually blacked out. The palpitations lasted for at least 10 minutes, and my pulse was so irregular and so fast that I could not count it. I went home and slept from three o'clock in the afternoon until nine that evening.

The next two days I still felt totally exhausted and slept all day, but the day after I decided I had to go back to work. I stayed at work all morning, but I felt so tired that I had to go home for lunch. Once there, I fell asleep and did not wake up until 4 p.m. (In case you are wondering what sort of job I had, I worked at a health centre in south-west London, where I was school nursing sister, did annual health surveys on the children and taught them sex education.)

The next three days were the same, and then the following day things got worse. I was at work when I started to feel very faint. I had palpitations and collapsed. A doctor was sent for, my pulse

1

was rapid and irregular, and I slept on a couch at work before being driven home later in the afternoon.

I slept all the next day before finally getting up at supper time. I still felt giddy, disorientated and confused. I rested all the next couple of days, as it was the weekend, but when I went back to work on the Monday the same thing happened. I collapsed again. The fatigue was dreadful – I could not even brush my hair, I felt so exhausted. The palpitations started again, and a friend took me to the doctor's surgery, where I was sent to the hospital for an ECG. It was normal. Even so, I felt so dizzy I could not focus at all – in fact, I felt so ill I thought I would die.

12 June: I slept all day, felt dizzy and first hot and then cold. Had tingles in my hands and feet and head and numbness in my legs. My vision was blurred, and I couldn't stand having the television on – the noise made me feel even worse. Every time I got out of bed I fell flat on my face.

13 June: Saw the doctor at the local hospital, and he gave me Stemitil for the dizziness and Amiodarone 200mg to settle my heart rhythm.

14 June: Rested all day. The fatigue is appalling. I have never felt so tired – it is as if my brain won't work at all.

15 June: Palpitations again. It frightens my children so much, because the palpitations show in my neck. My eyes look as though they have receded into my head, and I have this dreadful pallor. My eyes are excruciatingly painful, and everything I look at seemed to quiver.

16 June: I got up, but the palpitations started again, and I fell down the stairs. I had a terrible headache, my eyes could not focus, and I had an awful pain in the chest. I lay on the sofa and had palpitations from 9 a.m. to 6 p.m. I had extreme facial pallor, it looked like my eyes had receded into my head, and I felt like death. It was so frightening – the children thought I was having a heart attack.

17 June: The doctor came again and merely told me to rest.

17–26 June: I was too ill to get up. I just could not stay awake. I had nausea, vertigo and ringing in my ears. In addition, my hands, feet and head tingled, and my glands became very enlarged. I had a ticket for the centre court at Wimbledon, but there was no way I could go – I had to give it away.

For the next three to four weeks I stayed at home and rested. I felt incredibly sleepy, all day and all night. I hoped things would improve, but they did not. I felt constantly exhausted – every single thing I did exhausted me. It was absolutely the most I could do to summon up the energy to wash my face or brush my hair.

23 July: Went to see a doctor at Queen Mary's, Roehampton. He diagnosed post-viral fatigue syndrome. He was a consultant cardiologist, and he brought in his students to see me, because he said I was a classic case and had all the symptoms that would enable anyone to make a clinical diagnosis of ME. He was very nice and very kind and said he was very sorry but he could not recommend anything.

24 July – 9 August: I stayed at home and tried to get as much rest as possible. Basically I stayed in bed and only got up in order to go to the bathroom. If I tried to go downstairs I would fall over and have palpitations. My daughter, who was 16, took over the running of the house and did everything.

Then my mother came to look after me, but it was difficult, because what tired me most of all was having a conversation. Any mental effort made me really tired. If I got the slightest bit exhausted, the palpitations would start again, and I would feel desperately ill. So I just had to cut conversations short.

10 August: I went as a passenger in the car when my son took a friend to Heathrow and suddenly had horrific symptoms. Vertical railings flashing by made my brain feel scrambled. I felt confused and very anxious.

11 August: Dose of Amiodarone cut in half by doctor.

12 August: Palpitations returned with a vengeance and lasted for two hours.

4 September: I struggled in to work again, for the first time for a couple of months. I felt very tired and couldn't concentrate at all. I ached all over, couldn't remember things – I felt worse as the day wore on. So I had to go home again. By the time I got there, I had fallen over several times and bruised my legs. I could not talk properly and had an excruciating headache.

11 September: Cut the Amiodarone down to 100mg again.

14 September: Chest very painful, can't breathe properly, pain over right shoulder blade excruciating. Palpitations last over one-and-a-half hours.

19 September: Saw the doctor, and he said that, if everything settles down and I have no problems, then there is no need to see him again. If I do have problems, then come and see him again on 12 December. 'You play tennis,' he says, 'but if the cardiac arrhythmia happens again, go straight to Casualty, have an ECG and ask to see me earlier than December.'

25 September: Another awful relapse. Excruciating muscle pain and extreme exhaustion. I can't remember anything, and I can't even watch TV or read the paper. Even my hearing is strange. My legs are so wobbly, I fall over if I attempt to stand up out of bed. How many more symptoms can I get?

30 September: I feel so poorly today, I am so tired, I haven't got the energy to stroke my cat. My muscles are so excruciatingly painful that if I move my arms the muscles in my forearm go into spasm. I can't straighten my legs, because the spasms in my calf muscles are so excruciatingly painful. My headache is so bad that I have to keep my eyes closed and keep the sheet over my head because I can't bear the light in my bedroom but haven't got the energy to get up and draw the curtains.

1 October: I feel so exhausted, I can't move my body away from a crease in the sheet, and I haven't got enough energy to move a pillow. The muscle spasms and twitching of the muscles just get worse and worse. They fascinate my children because they can watch them. I can't swallow properly, the back of my throat is so dry. I can't get downstairs at all. My daughter has taken over and does everything.

11 November: I went out with a friend. I want to enjoy myself but feel so low. My friend thought I looked so ill I would die and a puff of wind would knock me over. I can't walk for more than 20 or 30 yards without the muscles in my calves going stiff – it is like trying to walk with lead shoes! I collapsed in the street and had to sit down in a café. Everyone stared.

17 November: I saw my GP. I needed Flagyl tablets for cystitis. I felt ill, with wobbly legs and upset stomach. I was sent to a psychotherapist, who said she thought that 'You have a little man sitting on your shoulder who always tells you to do things perfectly'. If I went to her once a week for two years, she said, she would help me to get rid of him!

I went home and felt angry that she did not realise I was so physically ill. I have been ill for 25 weeks now and feel worse and worse.

28 November: Another terrible relapse. I can't get downstairs because my legs are too weak. I keep trying but fall over, even if I have my daughter to lean on.

2 December: My GP called, as I feel like death and can't eat because of the nausea. I have mouth ulcers, I can't straighten my knees at all, my neck is so stiff, my feet and left side of my lips are totally numb, my head is so bad I can't focus, I am vomiting again. The doctor prescribed Indocid 50mg.

4 December: The doctor came again. I am so exhaused, I can hardly talk. I can't think or focus. In fact, it feels like I'm too exhausted even to breathe. My muscles ripple on their own without my moving my limbs. I feel drugged and poisoned, and every time I eat I feel worse. Quinine 300mg prescribed. Stopped taking the Flagyl tablets as a friend looked up Flagyl in a medical dictionary and noticed it should not be prescribed to people with central nervous system disorders. So it may be the Flagyl that has given me this relapse.

12 December: I saw a doctor at the hospital, and he said I had endogenous depression. I felt ill and exhausted on the way there, but I refused to have a wheelchair, because I was determined I would walk into the out-patients' department. I can't stand drawing attention to myself. The doctor told the students I was a typical case of ME and told me about the ME Association. When I got home, I collapsed into bed and felt terrible. I started Bolvidon 20mg tonight for the 'depression'. I am not depressed but will take them to prove that I want to get better – maybe they will help.

20 December: I have *got* to keep things going, for the children's sake. I am so worried about my daughter – she is only 16 years old and has been doing all the cooking, cleaning and shopping and looking after me. That is no life for a young girl. I must encourage her to go out at weekends. I ordered a microwave over the 'phone. It will save her time with the cooking.

22 December: The microwave arrived but I was too exhausted to go downstairs and see it.

23 December: I have had four weeks of feeling really ill now – probably as bad as I was at the beginning. No palpitations, but many more different symptoms. My lovely brother came up from Somerset to fetch us for Christmas. Spent four days with him and his family. They were so supportive and kind. Our friends have been with Christmas presents, but I feel too tired to open them. I can't use my arms they are too exhausted. I feel drugged. I think bread and Christmas cake and pudding give me a lift, and then I feel worse.

11 January 1987: Snow everywhere. I feel so cold, I can't get warm at all. The electric blanket is on high, but I can't get warm. My hands and feet are the coldest of all. I have had nine relapses now. What am I doing wrong? Talking exhausts me and makes my muscles ache. These anti-depressants do not seem to be helping at all. I think they make me feel less able to concentrate.

5

29 January: Admitted to National Hospital for Nervous Diseases. Lots of tests. EMV test the worst – it was so excruciating having an electric current through the muscles. I sobbed and sobbed, it was so painful I could not stop crying. The technician told me to stop making a fuss – all the staff had had the test done, and it did not hurt them. That night I was awake all night with muscle twitching in the arm they had tested. I felt ill and confused.

4 February: Sent to a physiotherapist at the National Hospital. I told them that physical exercise made me worse but merely got a scathing look from the physiotherapist. I tried my best but collapsed. I had to lie down on the couch. There was no apology from the therapist – she told me to walk back to the ward when I felt better.

5 February: I had a relapse in the hospital. I was talking to a visitor and then went pale and clammy and lost consciousness momentarily while lying in bed. I have had excruciating pains in the muscles since the shocks and needles through the muscles. I have co-operated but will never let anyone treat me like that again. I feel hot, then cold. Great discomfort in chest – feel as if my heart will stop, as it beats quickly and then misses a beat. All my joints are painful, and the glands in my neck are really enlarged.

16 February: Went to an ME meeting in SW7. Learnt such a lot. It was so good to talk to people who know exactly what you are experiencing. They all seem be to like me – work hard and are very sporty.

18 March: Started taking vitamins. They were sent from Lamberts and are all hypoallergenic – i.e. sugar-and yeast-free and free from all extras.

3 April: I had begun to realise that if the doctors could not help me, I must help myself. A very good friend of mine who had given me a tremendous amount of support brought me a copy of a book called *Candida Albicans: Is Yeast Your Problem?* by Leon Chaitow. Because I still couldn't read properly she underlined important passages for me and I realised that because of the white coating on my tongue and my problems with digestion I probably did have Candida. She went to the local health food store and bought me all the vitamins and probiotics such as lactobacillus that are recommended by the author. I also started to eliminate yeast from my diet. This made a dramatic difference – just stopping eating bread. The indigestion and gas subsided quite a lot within a fortnight. I also started to eat large quantities of live yoghurt and after three weeks the coating on my tongue was disappearing and I did not feel as confused and drowsy as I had done.

I also started taking zinc, vitamin C, vitamin A and selenium (all of which strengthen the immune system), vitamin B complex and *Lactobacillus Acidophilus*. And I was very strict about sticking to a yeast-free diet. I also cut all sugar out of my diet completely. I began to feel slightly better. I still felt depressed and weak but at least I had the energy to go downstairs and I felt especially pleased that I was able to wash up my own breakfast things. I thought that was a massive achievement after so many weeks of feeling so dreadful.

4 April: Started nystatin. I have applied for mobility allowance as I can only walk about 50 yards before the muscles in my calves go into spasm and I am forced to sit or lie down.

13 April: Went to Brighton for the day and enjoyed the fresh air on the beach. Felt so happy to be with a friend.

14 April: Why do I always have to pay for having a nice day? Another relapse. Perhaps I did too much.

10 May: Am 44 years old today. How painful, I feel 80. But at least I don't look it, thank goodness. Five weeks on nystatin now and a little energy is returning. I had forgotten what energy was. Now I find I have a little as long as I don't use it up too quickly. There only seems to be enough to do one thing like a little gardening – then I'm exhausted again. I must learn to pace myself.

26 May: Went to my son's parent-teachers' meeting. I rested for days so that I could make it but then was so light-headed when I got there that I couldn't concentrate. When I got home I tried to remember what had been said but I had forgotten almost all of it but thank goodness the friend who took me had made a note of the relevant remarks.

27 May: I was examined by the DHSS doctor for mobility allowance. He measured my calf muscles which appear to have wasted or maybe it's because I'm getting thin. There's very little muscle tone. I couldn't stand up without falling over.

4 July: I have been asked to resign my nursing sister's post. I feel so sad. I was paid six months' full salary and six month's half salary. I have no nursing pension as I always needed all my salary to pay for the children's school fees. What am I going to do now? I have tried so hard to get better and go back to work and it has caused 17 relapses so far.

9 July: A month ago I had a five-hour glucose tolerance test at University Hospital as I wondered if I was hypoglycaemic. It was positive. So I have been learning to eat little and often instead of three meals a day. This has made a big difference.

17 October: ME meeting at my house. This was at my suggestion as I couldn't get to the meetings at Hampstead or Gloucester Road. I find it so difficult to concentrate and keep awake. I wish I was as articulate as I used to be – I cannot say what I'm thinking properly.

18 October: I'm on lamb, potatoes and Perrier water prior to my third EPD injection. It's nine weeks since my last one. Have vomited twice and had to stop the taxi on the way to the hospital. The driver thinks I'm a real pain. I can see that!

31 October: Went out to dinner to an Italian restaurant. Had black-out and palpitations again. I thought I was going to die I felt so floppy. Frightened everyone around me. I don't know how I managed to walk up the stairs to the car. I was so confused I couldn't talk.

3 November: I noticed I began to get very sensitive to perfume. So when my daughter Amanda went out for the evening she would not put any scent on until she was outside the front door. Then she would push the bottle in its carton back through the letterbox. It affected me in a very dramatic way. My chest would feel as if it was tightening and it would seem to fold inwards so that I couldn't inhale properly and couldn't get enough air into my lungs. Even if someone came into the house wearing perfume it would really affect me – they didn't actually have to spray it on while they were indoors. Fresh air spray was also a problem – and furniture polishes. Fresh air spray was the worst.

One day I got off a train at Waterloo Station and I sat on the only available seat on the station to rest. Sitting next to me was a man who smelt very strongly of aftershave and it affected me so badly that I couldn't breathe properly and I collapsed. I fell off the seat and completely passed out because of this overwhelming smell.

19 February 1988: I am beginning to feel better from the EPD injections but I'm still pretty bad. I tell everyone I feel better as it saves explanations. I lie to people on the phone and say I'm up and about when in fact I can't get out of bed.

29 February: I'm learning a lot about ME on the radio and on TV. I still can't walk very far without great pain. I can have outings as long as I rest for days before and days afterwards. I can have

8

friends for lunch if I can rest for days afterwards. I don't tell any of them this as I'm afraid it will put them off.

1 May: Have had the house rewired. The noise made me feel awful and I can't rest properly in the afternoons. I find it essential to sleep for two to three hours in the afternoons. If I don't I can't keep going. If I *have* to go out in the afternoon, I need to stay in bed all morning and go to bed about 8 p.m. that evening.

23 May: My sixth EPD injection and I'm really beginning to improve. My allergies to household sprays and perfume and my sensitivity to strong smells have lessened considerably.

September 1988: Thanks to my wonderfully patient family and friends I feel I'm coming through this devastating disabling illness. How they have put up with the demands it has made on their lives I don't know. I feel the children have been cheated out of a healthy mother when as teenagers they needed one who was not 80 per cent disabled. However, I did appreciate the time I have had to reflect on my life and put things in perspective much more. How low on one's survival list I have found material things rate. When one has to exist from hour-to-hour, how precious life is. Until all the energy was taken away from me I certainly did not realise what a precious commodity it is.

These excerpts have been taken from Angela's diary between 1986 and 1988. I first met her at an ME support group, by which time, with the aid of a great deal of rest, many nutritional supplements and EPD (which will be discussed later in the book), she was considerably better. She does not have to stay in bed all day but she does rest for at least two-and-a-half hours every afternoon. She is careful about what she eats and even more careful about what she undertakes. Her case shows just how bad the symptoms of ME can be and how doctors seem to be able to do little about them. It shows also that if patients come to learn a great deal about the disease – and about health – they can find ways to alleviate the symptoms and regain control of their life.

2 How ME Hit the Headlines

Just two-and-a-half years ago the words *myalgic encephalo-myelitis* were unknown to the large majority of lay people and even the large majority of doctors.

But today there can be few people who have not heard of ME, or Yuppie 'flu, or post-viral fatigue syndrome, as it is sometimes called. ME has captured the imagination of the media and the public, and this interest all started on 1 June 1986 when one person decided to tell her story to the world.

That person was Sue Finlay. She told *The Observer* newspaper of her four-year battle to get treatment, even a diagnosis, for a disease that left her so fatigued she could not do the ironing, walk 50 yards, climb a flight of stairs. So tired she could not stand, or sit, or brush her hair, or clean her teeth, stir the soup or bring in the milk. A disease that rendered her constantly exhausted, irritable, weepy and depressed; that gave her aching joints, occasional palpitations, deteriorating eyesight, no appetite and a constant 'not quite right' tummy.

She wrote of the struggle with doctors who diagnosed her condition as 'nerves' and dosed her to the hilt with anti-depressants, tranquillizers and pain killers. She wrote of repeated blood tests and biopsies that all proved negative and prompted the doctors to suggest visits to the psychiatrist and more anti-depressants.

Sue Finlay's account of her illness immediately struck a chord. *The Observer* received 14,000 letters asking for a fact sheet about the disease. The ME Association, which was mentioned in the article received a flood of letters. Most of the correspondents had recognised their own symptoms from Sue Finlay's description. Many of them had a disease that defied the medical profession.

Doctors were baffled by the bewildering array of symptoms. They did not seem to fit any disease mentioned in the medical textbooks. And because the major symptom was fatigue doctors were not just baffled, they were suspicious. Fatigue, they knew from their training, could be a symptom of anaemia, pregnancy, diabetes, anorexia, glandular fever, hepatitis, heart disease, tuberculosis, hypothyroidism or Addison's disease and more. But if tests for all these conditions proved negative, what then? The medical textbooks all say much the same thing: when a physical cause cannot be found for fatigue an emotional one should be looked for. So doctors suspected an emotional cause and, as a result, many patients were dismissed as hypochondriacs, hysterics, or suffering from nerves or stress. But dismissing these patients from the surgery had not cured them; they kept on coming back.

After *The Observer* article other areas of the media started to take notice. Early in 1987, two women's glossy magazines, *Elle* and *Vogue*, carried features on the disease. Then the daily newspapers and the other Sundays carried features and on the radio *Medicine Now* ran a piece on ME.

A year after her original article, Sue Finlay told *The Observer* in a follow-up story how her condition had improved with the help of an anti-yeast diet and the drug nystatin that keeps infections of the fungus *Candida albicans* under control. Her first article had prompted a huge interest and she was now getting 200 letters a week from sufferers all over the UK.

'A year ago I would not have believed I could have the strength to cope with this, nor would I have believed so many people could be so ill and so desperate,' she said.

The discovery of the huge scale of misery prompted constructive anger. She decided to set up the ME Action Campaign to get the illness recognised by all doctors and the Department of Health, and to collect information through questionnaires, on the causes, symptoms and self treatment for the disease.

She said: 'I wrote the article when I was very ill myself and very angry. I had been told for years there was nothing physically wrong with me and that my debility and muscle fatigue . . . were all in the mind. I am still angry, not for myself, since my condition is greatly improved, but for all the other people being fobbed off with tranquillizers and sleeping pills.'

Sue Finlay accused the medical profession of not having the courage to face up to the disease. But there was a handful of doctors who recognised the seriousness of this condition and were trying to do something about it. One of these was Professor James Mowbray, professor of immunopathology at St Mary's Hospital in London. He was certain ME had an organic cause and was working on a diagnostic test that could be used by all doctors.

All ME sufferers must have been elated by the news in January 1988 that a specific blood test for ME had been perfected by Professor Mowbray. This would surely prove they had a real disease. But it was not that simple. Although the national newspapers reported that Mowbray had discovered a test for ME, in fact the test was for antibodies to enteroviruses. (We discuss this further in Chapter 4.) It was hardly conclusive because only 51 per cent of ME sufferers had positive results. And, as Mowbray pointed out, patients could have a negative result and still have ME. But it was a start. ME sufferers queued up for the test in their droves, anxious to prove to their GPs, their family, their friends, their employers, that they did indeed have a real, organic, disease.

The news from Mowbray's laboratory heightened the attention given to ME. But at the same time something happened that was to fuel the public interest even more. Clare Francis, author and former round-the-world yachtswoman, went public. She told of a battle with ME that had left her mind reduced to porridge and of a fatigue so profound she could barely climb the stairs.

'A week of vague flu-like symptoms developed into a fatigue so profound that I could barely climb the stairs. Even the effort of brushing my hair left me exhausted for hours. Weeks of rest and endless sleep did nothing to alleviate the fatigue. Other symptoms included vertigo, ringing in the ears, blurred vision, and a neck that felt as if it had been trapped in a vice. But these paled by comparison with the electrical storm in my brain – I literally couldn't think straight. I felt drugged, hungover, stupefied. An hour's writing reduced my thoughts to porridge and my speech to *non-sequiturs*. Worst of all a shutter had come down between me and the world: all sense of reality vanished.'

The decision to go public was a brave one and must have helped many people with ME. Here was a person, in the public eye, who was prepared to declare herself ill with a disease that doctors could not agree was real and that had no known cure. She became a Patron of the ME Action Campaign and its trustees decided to fight for recognition and support from the Government. They enlisted the help of Jimmy Hood, MP for Clydedale, who presented a Private Member's Bill under the ten-minute rule to the House of Commons on 23 February 1988. This Bill, the Myalgic Encephalomyelitis Bill was:

'A Bill to require an annual report to Parliament on progress made in investigating the causes, effects, incidence and treatment of the illness myalgic encephalomyelitis.'

The House voted in favour of hearing the Bill but time ran out in that session of Parliament and the Bill was never introduced. But it mattered not. A great deal of publicity was generated about ME and at last it was on the road to being recognised as an organic disease. Jimmy Hood said the importance of publicity for ME had been brought home to him by a telephone call from a woman sufferer.

'She told me she had decided to commit suicide that very morning and then heard an announcement that there was to be a radio programme on the subject of ME. Just hearing the news that somebody was doing something about ME was enough to change her mind.'

That was not the end of the story. ME was not a disease that was confined to Britain; from all over the world there came stories of sufferers and their difficulties in getting a diagnosis from their doctors.

From New Zealand, where there is a high incidence of the disease, there came news of 'Tapanui 'flu' named after a township in the South Island where there had been an epidemic. An active sufferers group in New Zealand, ANZMES (Australian and New Zealand ME Sufferers) was in close contact with the British ME Association and they kept each other informed of the latest developments.

In the United States suddenly everyone was talking about Yuppie 'Flu, so called because it seemed only to afflict young, high achievers. Among the US medical profession Yuppie 'Flu quickly became known as Chronic Epstein Barr Virus (CEBV) since reasearchers originally connected it with the Epstein Barr virus, one of the viruses in the Herpes group.

Incline, a fashionable ski resort in Nevada, reported at least two hundred cases among the small, resident, community. All were diagnosed by one general practitioner Dr Paul Cheney, who had the sense to listen to his patients' wide variety of symptoms and the determination to try and make some sense of them.

Back in Britain, two television programmes on ME were transmitted within one week of each other. The first probably did more to set back the cause of ME sufferers than anything that had been written or said since 1970 when ME was first dismissed as hysteria (more about that in Chapter 3). A *Where There's Life* programme hosted by Dr Miriam Stoppard interviewed sufferers and an expert in immunology and concluded that this debilitating disease was a bandwagon onto which any tired, depressed, hypochondriac could crawl.

The only doctor invited to talk on the show was Dr Richard Powell, consultant immunologist at the Queen's Medical Centre in Nottingham. He told the audience that eight out of ten people claiming to have ME would be cured by a good night's sleep. To anyone who knew anything about ME it appeared that Dr Powell had little experience of the illness himself. It turned out that he had been recommended to the programme makers as an ME expert by the British Medical Association. The BMA is often asked to provide information about a variety of diseases but it is the responsibility of every journalist or television researcher who uses this service to check that they are indeed getting the experts in the field. This was obviously not done by the *Where There's Life* team.

The people interviewed on the programme had obviously not been chosen on the basis of their symptoms but probably more to support what seemed to be the central theme of the programme – that people who think they have ME are 'suffering from life', or, in other words, experiencing depression.

A storm of protest followed. Clare Francis, supported by Jimmy Hood, demanded that the Independent Broadcasting Authority should put pressure on the *Where There's Life* producers to make another programme presenting a more balanced view of the disease and include ME sufferers and experts who had actually worked with ME patients. Clare Francis and another sufferer were given the chance to air their views on the *Right to Reply* programme.

The second television programme was a *Horizon* special on BBC2. Its main aim was to tackle the central dilemma of ME – is it an organic or a psychological disease? It was a well-balanced appraisal and included all the ME specialists and four sufferers, all at different stages of their disease. There was no escaping the final message: doctors have no answer for ME so patients must try to help themselves. This is the reason we have written this book. Doctors and the media continue to argue about the cause of ME. In reality that is not so important. What is important is that an estimated 200,000 people in Britain have an illness for which there is no recognised cure. While the experts wrangle there are people suffering. It is up to patients to find out as much about ME as possible – to find their own cure.

This book is designed to help you understand ME, its possible cause, and to explain how we think you can get better. Although there is no one cure for ME, there are many things that sufferers can do to relieve their symptoms and to speed recovery. We have drawn on the worlds of both orthodox and alternative (or complementary) medicine and found good things in both. We have analysed questionnaires sent in by hundreds of sufferers to find out how ME has changed your lives and show how you can cope with these changes.

First, however, we will look at the history of ME because that is crucial, not just for an understanding as to what might cause it, but for an understanding of why many doctors thought – and indeed still think – it has a psychological cause.

3 A History of ME: when did it first occur? A brief account of the major outbreaks. Why it was nonsense to label it hysteria

With all the attention that has been give to ME in the past two years you might be forgiven for thinking it is a new disease. But the illness has probably been with us since time began: masquerading under different names, going unrecognised or being mistaken for something else.

Dr Darrel Ho-Yen, immunologist for Northern Scotland who has seen many cases of ME, believes it has existed for as long as there have been viral infections and that would seem to make sense. Recognition of a disease depends on documentation and illnesses are unlikely to get documented where cases occur sporadically in ones and twos. Epidemics are a different matter. They are reported in medical journals and so it is to the epidemics that we must look to find the history of ME.

The first major epidemic in the UK was in 1955 at London's Royal Free Hospital. It was this that first brought ME into the public spotlight and it was to send the medical profession into turmoil and confusion. Doctor was set against doctor in the debate that is still continuing today to decide whether ME is a psychological disease or a 'real' organic one.

A description of the outbreak in the *British Medical Journal* of 19 October 1957 gives a concise account from the medical team charged with caring for patients affected:

> On July 13th 1955 a resident doctor and a ward sister on the staff of the Royal Free Hospital were admitted to the wards with an obscure illness. By July 25th more than 70 members of the staff were similarly affected and it was plain that there was in the hospital an epidemic of a highly infectious nature producing, among other things, manifestations of the central nervous system. Because of the threat to

16

patients and because of the large numbers of nurses involved, the hospital closed on that date and remained closed until October 5th. By that time the epidemic was almost over although sporadic cases appeared up to November 24th.

Between July 13th and November 24th, 292 members of the medical, nursing, auxiliary medical, ancillary and administrative staff were affected by the illness and of these 255 were admitted to hospital; 37 nurses were looked after at home or admitted to other hospitals from their home. It is remarkable that although the hospital was full at the time of the epidemic only 12 patients who were already there developed the disease.

The earliest symptoms in the Royal Free epidemic were malaise and headache sometimes accompanied by depression and constantly changing emotional state. This was often accompanied by other symptoms including sore throat, headaches, nausea, abdominal pain, vomiting, diarrhoea. During the second and third weeks most of the patients developed quite severe symptoms. The report in the *British Medical Journal* describes them as suffering severe pain in the neck, back or limbs, dizziness, blurred vision, tinnitus, vertigo.

In addition, 74 per cent of the 200 patients described in the report developed neurological symptoms. Some patients suffered partial paralysis of the facial muscles. Some developed blurred near vision because the eye muscles had become weak. Some patients were unable to swallow because of weak muscles and they had to be fed with a tube. The slightest attempt to move the limbs caused severe pain in some patients. A few became completely paralysed while others lost the use of their arms or legs through weakness, some suffered bladder problems and could not urinate. Many reported spontaneous pain in their limbs.

Despite the plethora of symptoms and despite extensive investigations, Dr Melvin Ramsay, consultant in infectious diseases at the Royal Free at the time of the outbreak, was unable to find any virus or other organism that could possibly be responsible for the epidemic. However, he was certain 'Royal Free disease', as it was known then, was not unique to the Royal Free. Throughout 1955, '56 and '57 sporadic cases of a similar illness were admitted to the hospital from the general community. In May 1955 patients had begun to turn up at the Royal Free with muscular weakness. At first it was thought they had polio but in most cases the polio virus could not be isolated. In 1955, 16 cases were admitted from the general community of north London, in 1956 there were 18 cases and in 1957 another 19. But it was the cases at the Royal Free that had made national newspaper headlines.

Dr Ramsay believed the Royal Free outbreak had arisen 'as a direct result of a nest of sporadic cases over a large area of north London which had been present since the Spring of 1955'.

He and a colleague described the first eight cases of this 'nest' in *The Lancet* of 26 May 1956 and a further 34 cases of this 'new entity' were reported in *The Lancet* 18 months later on 14 December 1957. The dominant feature was muscle fatigability: 'Following even a minimal degree of physical exertion there could be delays of three to five days before muscle power was restored.'

Patients also reported 'coldness of the extremities, hypersensitivity to climatic change and a ghastly facial pallor often first noticed by friends or relatives'. Another major feature was cerebral involvement. Dr Ramsay reported that many of the patients had impaired memory and concentration. Their emotions were unpredictable and constantly changing and they had vivid dreams, often in colour. Complaints of not being able to tolerate loud noises were interspersed with periods of normal hearing or even deafness.

The patients' symptoms conformed to the same pattern. 'All cases, whether with or without neurological involvement, showed proneness to fatigue after physical exertion and by this time it was clear that this could persist for weeks or months after the initial attack.'

Other Outbreaks

The Royal Free epidemic is the one that has attracted most attention in this country but, in fact, epidemics have occurred in many other parts of the world. Around 52 outbreaks of ME have occurred to date – all of them marked by muscle fatigue and a legacy of physical incapacity.

In 1934, Los Angeles was the scene of an outbreak involving 198 members of medical and nursing staff at the city's County General Hospital that was an almost exact precursor of the Royal Free outbreak some 21 years later. The initial symptoms of the

Los Angeles outbreak were similar to poliomyelitis with local-ised muscle weakness in 80 per cent of the patients, but none of the muscle wasting that occurs in polio. Muscle pain, tenderness, loss of concentration, lapses of memory, sleep disturbances, emotional lability with hysterical episodes and fatigue on walking short distances were a prominent feature. Six months after the epidemic, 55 per cent of the patients were still off duty. Sporadic cases of the disease were being reported right up to 1965 around the Los Angeles area.

Switzerland was the scene of the next two recorded epidemics and they are of interest because they both occurred in exclusively male communities – battalions of the Swiss army. Many critics of the organic theory of ME have said that because the disease seems to affect women more than men it has a psychological origin. Women are alleged to suffer from hysteria and depression more than men and that is why they are thought by some to make up the majority of ME sufferers. But just to disprove this theory, in 1937, 130 soldiers in a group of 930 went down with a systemic illness that developed into encephalomyelitis with mild muscle weakness. Two years later 73 cases of 'abortive poliomyelitis' were reported in men from a battalion of soldiers arriving from an area where polio was rife. Once again muscle fatigability, sometimes persisting for more than a year, was a major feature.

Eleven years later in Iceland, patients from several districts around the town of Akureyri developed what was at first thought to be poliomyelitis; once again the disease was characterised by muscle fatigue. A follow-up study seven years later found that only 25 per cent of the patients had fully recovered. Many of the patients were still complaining of nervousness, abnormal muscle fatigue, muscle pain, insomnia and loss of memory. And Dr Betty Scott, the Finchley GP who has made a special study of the Iceland epidemic and has visited the country 14 times, says that of the nine Icelandic patients she has seen in the last two years –nearly 40 years after the epidemic – only one has completely recovered.

In Adelaide, Australia, an epidemic of poliomyelitis seemed to change direction to become an outbreak of ME. Between August 1949 and April 1951 700 cases of this unknown disease that seemed to mimic polio were admitted to hospital – the ratio of men to women was 1:1.

In New York State, in 1950, another outbreak of 'abortive poliomyelitis' was reported and named 'Iceland disease' because of its similarities with the 1948 Akureyri outbreak.

Back in London an outbreak of an infectious disease involving the central nervous system was described in *The Lancet* of 20 November 1952. Although the outbreak involved just 14 nurses, Dr Donald Acheson, a physician at the Middlesex Hospital and now the British Government's chief medical officer, thought it worth describing the cases because of their unusual features and similarity to other problematic epidemics that had occurred in previous years. Once again severe muscular pains affecting the back, limbs, abdomen and chest as well as muscle weakness and fatigue characterised the illness.

In 1955, the year of the Royal Free epidemic, another outbreak occurred bearing a remarkable similarity to what was happening in London. In Dalston, Cumbria the local GP was being swamped with cases, starting in February 1955 when there was an epidemic among the primary school children of the region that quickly spread to adults. By July, 233 children out of 1,675 children in the practice had gone down with this mysterious illness, an incidence of 14 per cent. The main features of the disease had an almost predictable similarity with other epidemics of ME and over the next few years around 20 per cent of the patients had relapsed.

Another general community outbreak occurred between 1964 and 1966 in Finchley, north London. In all, 370 cases were seen by the GP at the time, Dr Betty Scott, who took very careful case histories and would not diagnose ME unless most of the characteristic symptoms were present: low-grade fever, headache, blurred vision, muscular weakness that was unrelieved by rest, emotional lability, insomnia, frequency or retention of urine.

Dr Scott still lives in Finchley and, although she retired as a GP ten years ago, she still sees some of her original ME patients.

'Nearly all my patients were intelligent,' she says. 'Very few of them were not. If you look carefully at their case histories it is obvious that overwork was the precipitating factor.'

The Hospital for Sick Children at Great Ormond Street was home to the next epidemic when 145 staff went down with the disease between August 1970 and January 1971. The doctors who reported it in the medical press said: 'Ten or 11 of the commonest symptoms were almost identical with those reported in the Royal Free outbreak in 1955.' But they had trouble with one symptom and omitted it from their list because they found it very hard to quantify – that symptom was rapid fatigability reported on exercise. None of the children were affected during the outbreak although some had been admitted to the hospital beforehand with symptoms that were similar to the disease.

The next three outbreaks all occurred in Scotland and were interesting because of a new development: the discovery of raised antibodies to a virus called Coxsackie. In West Kilbride, Ayrshire between 1980 and 1983, 22 patients were seen with suspected ME. All had extreme exhaustion, particularly after exercise, but it also followed emotional or mental strain. Blood tests revealed that 82 per cent of the patients had raised antibody levels to Coxsackie B Virus.

The West Kilbride outbreak prompted a GP in Balfron, Stirlingshire to take another look at some of the patients in his practice who had protracted illnesses similar to those in Ayrshire. Once again, raised antibody levels to Coxsackie B were found in the patients suspected of having ME. Another Scottish GP, in Helensburgh, re-examined his 'troublesome' patients and found that 47 per cent of the 81 suspected cases of ME had raised antibody levels of Coxsackie B virus.

The Disease in the Community
These epidemics of ME are very illuminating but what do they mean to the ordinary sufferer isolated alone in the community? Are epidemics of ME and the sporadic cases in the general population the same disease?

According to Dr Melvin Ramsay, who has had more experience of this disease than any other doctor, the epidemic ME and the endemic ME are one and the same. He says:

'ME is an endemic disease which is subject to periodic outbreaks of epidemic prevalence. Outbreaks such as those in Los Angeles and Iceland were undoubted epidemics with rapid case-to-case spread, but the outbreaks in north-west London in 1955 and Finchley in 1964 consisted of groups of sporadic cases with no history of known contact with infectious cases.'

Dr Ramsay collaborated with Dr Betty Scott after the 1964 epidemic in a study of more than 50 patients. None of them had been associated with an outbreak of the disease and their own doctors had virtually given up trying to help them. Dr Ramsay says:

'The patients whom Dr Scott and I saw came to us in a state of utter despair, their medical advisors finding themselves baffled by a medley of symptoms which they were unable to place into any recognisable category of disease.'

Many of these patients had been referred to neurologists who had not been able to do anything for them. They had also made their way to the psychiatrist's couch and Dr Ramsay recalls at least four psychiatrists who returned patients back to the GP with a note to the effect that they did not know what the patients were suffering from, but they were certainly not psychiatric cases.

Dr Ramsay's and Dr Scott's research revealed that the disease occurring in the community had a similar onset and progression to the epidemic forms and was probably the same disease. They also uncovered the depths of human misery that ME can cause. They found families split up through ME, people who committed suicide through ME, people who had to forfeit their careers through ME, people who could not look after their own children through ME.

The two doctors strove to convince the medical profession of the despair and hopelessness that ME can provoke in its victims. But then something happened that must have come as a terrible blow. Their work of 15 years was dismissed in just a few pages of one of the most prestigious medical journals in the country, for in 1970, two psychiatrists pronounced ME as nothing more than mass hysteria.

The psychiatrists, Dr McEvedy and Dr Beard, had studied the casenotes of the nurses involved in the Royal Free outbreak of 1955 and they reported in the *British Medical Journal* in 1970 that Royal Free disease was due to mass hysteria. They also attributed the outbreak among 14 nurses at the Middlesex Hospital in 1952 to mass hysteria. But they said the outbreaks in Los Angeles and others that were associated with poliomyelitis were not such 'pure examples' of mass hysteria.

McEvedy and Beard's hypothesis was seized on by the popular press of the day, including *Time* magazine, and seems to have been readily accepted as fact by the majority of the medical profession.

Dr Ramsay and his colleagues pointed out that 'while a diagnosis of hysteria had been seriously considered at the time of the outbreak, the occurrence of fever in 89 per cent, lymphadenopathy (swollen glands) in 79 per cent, of ocular palsy (paralysis of the eye muscles) in 43 per cent and of facial palsy (paralysed facial muscles) in 19 per cent rendered it quite untenable.' Dr Donald Acheson, who had reported the 1952 Middlesex Hospital outbreak in *The Lancet*, said he had ruled out a diagnosis of mass hysteria for similar reasons.

However no one seemed to pay any attention to these responses and McEvedy and Beard's hypothesis quickly became a 'fact'. It is worth pointing out that Dr McEvedy had a special interest in hysteria. In 1966 he had reported in the medical journals outbreaks of overbreathing among schoolchildren in Blackburn and Portsmouth, epidemics that were 'incompatible with an organic illness.' And, most important of all, patients from the Royal Free epidemic who were still suffering with relapses 15 years later were not examined by McEvedy and Beard, nor were any of the other patients involved in the outbreak.

Dr Ramsay admits that there may be an element of hysteria in some patients with ME. Emotional fluctuations appear in most accounts of the disease. But another characteristic of hysteria, hyperventilation or overbreathing, does not seem to occur. Dr Betty Scott, who reported the 1964 Finchley outbreak, said hyperventilation had never been observed in any of the 370 cases she examined. But hypoglycaemia (low blood-sugar levels) had been measured in many of the patients. Low blood sugar can cause fainting and could easily be mistaken for hysteria if it was not checked. Other symptoms which Dr Scott reported might be mistaken for hysteria were twitching muscles, rapid eye movements, dizziness and a markedly pale face.

The hysteria hypothesis had been considered as far back as 1938 but it had been discounted in the face of the overriding evidence of organic illness. In a report on the Los Angeles epidemic Dr Gilliam, the medical officer in charge, wrote:

'The emotional upsets are difficult to interpret. They vary in degree from relatively slight displays of irritability and impatience to violent dislikes of people and things formerly liked. A common type of upset takes the form of unprovoked bouts of weeping. The emotional upsets of a few people were undoubtedly hysterical but it would be manifestly erroneous to consider as hysteria the emotional instability associated with this illness in all the cases in which it was present.'

Another factor that would discount hysteria is that cases in the same household varied in the features and the course of the illness. Also in all the epidemics the illness was remarkably similar despite the variety of people and communities that were affected, making hysteria unlikely. The disease was consistent from outbreak to outbreak, in different countries in different years and different peoples. The emotional symptoms of ME –

depression, emotional lability, impaired memory and powers of concentration – are all consistent with an organic disease rather than the shallow, generally short-lived symptoms of hysteria. And hysteria does not explain the muscle weakness that occurred in all the outbreaks reported – or the fatigue after exercise.

Dr Scott wrote a letter to the *BMJ* in response to the McEvedy and Beard article. Her letter was sent with the backing of the Royal Free doctors and in it she said she had read the article with incredulity. 'It is my hope the views expressed by Drs McEvedy and Beard will not be taken seriously', she wrote, 'especially as the implied diagnosis of "hysteria" to a seriously ill patient can cause acute distress and prolong the illness indefinitely.' Now she calls their hypothesis 'scandalous. They did more damage to patients than you would believe possible.'

According to Dr Ramsay, it was the blinkered approach of the medical profession in seizing on the idea of mass hysteria so readily that left a generation of doctors ignorant of this organic disease and a generation of ME sufferers in despair. Without the McEvedy and Beard hypothesis and the credence given to it it is probable that many sufferers would not have had to experience so many months or years of frustration in searching for a diagnosis. As Jimmy Hood said in the House of Commons, 'the greatest suffering of all is the anguish caused by misdiagnosis.'

It is noteworthy that in the 5 March 1988 issue of the *British Medical Journal* there appeared an article entitled 'Post-Viral Fatigue Syndrome: Time for a New Approach'. In it three psychiatrists, Drs Anthony David, Simon Wessely and Anthony Pelosi, said: 'We have personal experience in the care and investigation of patients with the post-viral fatigue syndrome and are in no doubt about the genuineness and severity of the condition. Present controversy rests on a false dualism and an outdated separation of mind and body, and the shortcomings of these approaches are emphasised by increasing knowledge of the biological abnormalities in psychiatric disorders.'

In other words, doctors should not separate psychological and physical illnesses and should start treating the patient as a whole.

Summary

The history of ME can be summed up as follows. The first recorded major outbreak was the one in Los Angeles in 1934. At first it looked like polio but it didn't quite fit. Significantly, 54 per cent of the sufferers were still unable to return to work six months later. And 14 years later all the patients in a 21 patient study still had considerable symptoms. Then came the ones in Switzerland in two different army barracks which should have shown future generations of doctors that they were wrong in suspecting it was largely a female disease.

Then came Iceland and with it, unfortunately because it confused the issue, a new name 'Iceland disease'. It was followed by the outbreak in New York in 1949, the first in which doctors looked for evidence of the Coxsackie virus. Then came the epidemic at the Royal Free where, in spite of extensive virological testing, no virus was found. It was the largest outbreak yet, it caused a whole hospital to be closed down for three months and the following year *The Lancet* gave the disease a name: *Benign myalgic encephalomyelitis*.

Some of the Royal Free nurses were not much better in 1970 – fifteen years later – but when McEvedy and Beard wrote their article it seems they did not bother to check. McEvedy had previously examined outbreaks of illness he put down to hysteria and so it perhaps should not have been a surprise when he reached the same conclusion about the Royal Free. What is a surprise is that his appraisal was accepted so readily – and accepted as fact.

Throughout the 1970s, Ramsay's work was ignored and the excellent work of Peter Behan and other Scottish doctors in the early 1980s seems to have made little impact. The McEvedy and Beard hypothesis accounted for what can be looked back on as 'the dark ages of ME', a period between 1970 and, to all intents and purposes, 1986, in which patients who reported its symptoms to their doctor were for the most part treated with disbelief, scorn or derision, dismissed with tranquillizers or sent to a psychiatrist.

Now, in late 1988, comes perhaps the best evidence of all that the Royal Free epidemic should never have been attributed to hysteria. Of the nurses involved, 97 have just revealed to Dr Ramsay that 33 years later they still suffer from ME and have not recovered.

3a   A Note About Terms: ME, Post Viral Syndrome, Chronic Fatigue Syndrome

Much of the early confusions about ME was caused by the profusion of names appended to it, of which Royal Free Disease, Iceland Disease, benign myalgic encephalomyelitis, and neuro-myasthenia were just four. Now there is equal confusion about ME and post-viral fatigue syndrome. The latter, or PVS as it is sometimes called, is something many people get after a bout of influenza or other virus infection. It is not pleasant. The fatigue and listlessness can be considerable but it does go away, often after a few weeks, sometimes after several months. It rarely lasts more than a year.

PVS
What is confusing about PVS is that the symptoms can be the same as ME, but it is probably true to say that they are often fewer in number. Dr Ramsay is at present trying to get doctors to recognise the difference between PVS and ME. He thinks, and we agree, that this confusion is the major reason why many doctors are taking ME so lightly. They will tell patients: 'It's nothing more than a bit of post-viral syndrome.' Well, it is more: ME is a major illness and can last for many years. Sheila Neal, for example, one of the nurses who went down with ME during the Royal Free epidemic in 1955 is still unwell. As are 96 other Royal Free nurses. And there are many sufferers around today who contracted ME in the 1960s and 1970s and have made little recovery.

Chronic Fatigue Syndrome
In America ME was thought by some doctors to be caused by the Epstein Barr virus and was called CEBV (Chronic Epstein Barr Virus Syndrome). This theory has now largely been abandoned and scientists are hunting for the virus or viruses responsible. It is

possible that they will come round to Professor Mowbray's point of view that the culprits are enteroviruses. But in the meantime, just to make it even more confusing, they have come up with another name – Chronic Fatigue Syndrome.

Now, this is not a bad name for ME. It sums up the nature of the beast. Fatigue is what it is all about and the word 'chronic' makes it clear that the fatigue is not restricted to a post-viral illness. Unlike the phrase post-viral fatigue syndrome it includes all those cases of severe and chronic fatigue that were not preceded by a viral infection.

So Chronic Fatigue Syndrome is a sensible phrase and it is one that can be applied to all those people who have very real symptoms but do not have a positive response to Professor Mowbray's test for antibodies to enteroviruses. Sufferers who do not have a positive test should not feel bad about it. They should not fear that their symptoms are all in the mind after all. What they have is Chronic Fatigue Syndrome. It is not pleasant, it is very hard to get rid of, but we hope that by reading this book you will get some ideas about how to defeat it.

4 The Symptoms: have you got ME?

One of the most remarkable aspects of ME is the number and variety of symptoms its sufferers describe in addition to the basic one of overwhelming fatigue. For the person who is in the early stages of the illness it might seem incredible that such a wide range of symtoms could belong to just one disease. How is it that muscle fatigue, tinnitus, headaches, vertigo, mental confusion, stomach upsets, depression, irritability, inability to concentrate, sensitivity to temperature, pins and needles, blurred vision could possibly belong to the same illness? The answer to that question is still one of the big unknowns of ME.

What is known is that a diagnosis should not be made on the basis of one single symptom. All sufferers have a range of symptoms and if you have only one or two it is unlikely that you have ME. Each patient is different and each will have a number of symptoms and not necessarily the same ones that another sufferer has. However, there are a few that all sufferers will experience at some time during their illness.

The Onset of ME
ME has many different beginnings. Some people can trace it back to the time they had a bout of 'flu, or glandular fever or a respiratory infection. It may happen suddenly and without an apparent cause or it may come on slowly and gradually. There will be persistent and profound fatigue accompanied by a medley of symptoms. Most doctors will not make a diagnosis of ME until these have been present for at least six months. There are viral infections with similar symptoms that will disappear within three to six months, glandular fever, for instance. What marks out the ME patient is that recovery is prolonged or the patient suffers relapse after relapse, lulled in the intervening periods into thinking he or she may be getting better.

No one should be certain they have ME until the symptoms have lasted some time. Some people will declare they suffered ME after a bout of influenza, but the fatigue, malaise and lethargy that sometimes follows 'flu should more properly be called post-viral fatigue syndrome. This has many of the same symptoms as ME but the essential difference is that patients recover – usually within six months and almost always within a year.

It is this confusion of terms that has led to one of the myths about ME that is often propagated by doctors who are not very familiar with the disease. That is that patients will somehow get better automatically. One has only to look at the several hundreds of patient questionnaires we have scrutinised to see that this is not the case. Almost all are not better than they were two, five, seven or even ten and fifteen years previously. Post-viral fatigue syndrome will go away; ME or 'persistent' or 'chronic' fatigue syndrome probably will not. But it can be managed and with the right combination of therapies the symptoms can be very considerably reduced.

Fatigue
Extreme fatigue, both physical and mental, is the symptom that unites all ME sufferers. Every ME patient will recognise the enormous fatigue of this illness but the scale of the fatigue can sometimes be difficult to explain to doctors, family and friends. Most sufferers would agree that there is no word in the English language sufficient to describe the tiredness of ME.

American sufferer, Hillary Johnson, wrote in *Rolling Stone* magazine: 'One year four months ago I was in control of my career and life. Now my days are defined by an enigmatic disease that renders me profoundly fatigued and, at its worst, has left me unable to lift my toothbrush or remember my phone number.'

Another victim told of how on a trip to London she felt the strength drain from her legs before she could reach the Underground. She had to take refuge in a hotel for the night. Some patients are worse; they find it hard to climb even one flight of stairs.

Many diseases manifest themselves with fatigue as one of the symptoms, ME is unique in that the fatigue is made worse by exercise. Every ME patient could come up with copious examples of how exercise has affected their way of life. One of these is Nicky Spurgeon who, at the age of 22, was England's number four women's squash player. After contacting ME she could barely walk onto a squash court; five minutes of play reduced her legs to jelly.

One sufferer told of her husband's attempts to get her out into

29

the fresh air 'thinking a bit of exercise would do me good. It worked in completely the opposite way and I was in a state of virtual collapse by the end of the street.'

Dr Melvin Ramsay says, 'After moderate exercise from which a normal person would recover with nothing more than a good night's rest, an ME patient will require at least three to four days. After more strenuous exercise the period can be prolonged to two or three weeks.

'If, during this recovery period, there is a further expenditure of energy the effect is cumulative and this is responsible for the unrelieved sense of exhaustion and depression which characterises the chronic case.'

Some of the doctors involved in the virological studies of the three Scottish outbreaks described in Chapter 3 have studied this muscle fatigue in ME patients. Dr Peter Behan, Dr Wilhelmina Behan and Dr Eleanor Bell reported in the medical journal *Infectious Diseases* in October 1984 their study of 50 patients whose primary symptom was gross fatigue made worse on exercise.

Eighteen men and 32 women were included in the study and all had had the illness for an average of five years (the range being three months to 22 years). The researchers could find no evidence of muscle weakness in any of the muscle groups they examined after the patients had been resting. But if the patients were asked to squeeze a rubber ball attached to an ergometer for one minute there was marked muscle weakness that lasted for an hour.

Ten of the patients were asked to climb 40 steps and, in all of them, there was severe weakness of the legs, sometimes lasting up to three hours. Although the reasons for these abnormalities could not be explained by this study, the researchers said that an increased formation of lactic acid in the muscles or a decreased ability to metabolise normal amounts of lactic acid might explain the weakness.

Since then, analysis of the muscle fibres of ME patients using a technique called single fibre electromyography, has revealed that the majority display some abnormality in the muscles.

In Oxford, Professor George Radda has been using nuclear magnetic resonance to measure the chemical changes taking place in the muscles during exercise. His work has shown that weak muscles tend to burn up energy more quickly than normal muscles and this could explain why people with ME become tired so quickly.

Sometimes only one side of the body will be affected by muscle weakness, but if both sides are it is generally the side that is most used in daily activities that will be more severely affected. So in a right-handed person the muscles of the left hand and arm would be slightly stronger.

But physical fatigue is not the only tiredness that ME sufferers have to bear. Most report a mental fatigue that renders them unable to read a book or watch television or even listen to the radio. Many sufferers cannot even keep up with a normal conversation and for some the mental confusion is so bad they even use the phrase, 'mentally handicapped'.

A 39-year-old man, well-known in the 1970s for his dynamic running of a community organisation, describes his symptoms as 'Very up and down with no rhyme or reason for it. Optimistic most of the time but sometimes depressed and even suicidal. Sometimes not just mentally confused but totally disabled.'

Another sufferer, a woman fired from her job and divorced by her husband, says, 'Of all the things I have missed, I miss my mind the most.'

Other Symptoms Related to Fatigue
Many other symptoms suffered by ME patients can be related to muscle weakness, the most common are:

Blurred vision: In the reports of the ME epidemics blurred vision was a very common symptom and it is one that many patients report. The eye is a complex of muscles that adjust the lens so that we can see clearly. If the muscles of the eye become weak they will not adjust the lens to near and far vision and consequently the vision becomes blurred.

Dribbling: Sometimes the muscles that control the jaw become so weak that the mouth hangs open and the sufferer dribbles in his or her sleep.

Coldness of the Extremities and Sensitivity to Change of Temperature
Virtually every ME patient suffers coldness of the extremities and hypersensitivity to climatic change. A sudden drop in temperature may make normal people feel a little bit cold but ME sufferers will really shiver. It seems that their body finds it difficult to adapt. Cold hands and feet may result from impaired blood circulation and it is often relatives or friends who notice that the sufferer has a marked pallor on the days when he or she feels unwell.

General Malaise or 'Just Feeling Awful All the Time'

A wide variety of symptoms come into this category and many sufferers find it difficult to pinpoint just what it is that makes them feel constantly under par.

Jenny Culverwell must have summed up the feelings of many ME patients when she described her symptoms on Radio 4's *Woman's Hour*. ME crept up on her insidiously over some time. 'The thing that is so difficult to describe is this overpowering unwell sensation, the feeling of complete disorientation, sea sick, giddiness.'

Aches and Pains

Headache: a severe headache was often the first sign that something was wrong in the earlier outbreaks. Although probably not 'true' migraines, the headaches associated with ME can be extremely painful and 'migrainous' in nature – that is patients can only relieve the pain by sleeping it off.

Spontaneous muscle pains: these may occur anywhere in the body but particularly in the abdomen and in the limbs that are the weakest. Many patients report tingling or pins and needles, others tell of jerking limbs and muscle spasms or spontaneous twitches. A 30-year-old sufferer who has been ill for eight years describes 'hot rods of pain' shooting from her shoulders to finger tips and from her knees to her toes.

Ear and Eye Symptoms

There is a wide range of these.

Tinnitus: this is fairly common. This is a ringing or noise in the ears that is sometimes constant and sometimes comes and goes.

Sensitivity to noise: this is also a problem for sufferers. Not just traffic noise which can be offensive to everyone, but even more mundane noises such as the telephone or radio.

Sensitivity to light: this is also a common symptom and sufferers can only bear to be in a room when the curtains are drawn and the lights are off.

Vertigo: this happens particularly at the onset of ME and can be very frightening. Sometimes it is so severe that just a slight movement of the head can bring a flood of dizziness and the overwhelming feeling of being off-balance.

For Jenny Culverwell the vertigo was particularly severe: 'I can remember crossing a road several times to post a letter and on my way back stumbling to the wall. I was trying to use every ounce of effort in my body to control myself, to control my mind, to control my body from shaking . . . just to control myself to walk down the path so that I could lie on the floor inside my own home and not have to lie on the pavement.'

Mental Symptoms
There is no doubt that a good deal of the misery of ME is caused by changes of mood and emotional state that go hand in hand with physical symptoms. Some patients find it almost too much to bear when they break down in tears for no reason at all where previously they had rarely cried. Some are struck down by a black depression which is a common feature of ME. This can be one of the most dangerous aspects of the disease as it is all too easy to become swallowed up in a downward spiral of despair. The number of suicides as a direct result of ME is unknown but there have been at least eight cases that can probably be attributed to it. One victim documented by Dr Ramsay was a young man who had battled with ME for two years and whose mother also had the disease. When the 22-year-old went to university he found the reversal of sleep rhythms that ME had induced too much to bear and he took an overdose of a tranquillizer.

Sleep disorders are very common. Most ME patients sleep for long periods of time but do not feel fully rested when they wake up. As one sufferer says, 'When I wake up I feel so totally crippled for at least three-quarters of an hour that I have to take pain-killers.'

Other ME patients may find themselves waking at odd hours of the night and early morning and then falling asleep all day. A note of warning here: waking up early in the morning, every morning, can be a classic sign of depression and it is important for ME sufferers to be clear whether their early waking is due to ME or an underlying depression that has not been recognised.

Gastro-Intestinal Problems
Some of these problems may be related to food allergies that ME patients may develop (discussed in detail in Chapter 7). Diarrhoea or an upset stomach may recur from time to time and when this occurs together with pain in the abdomen it can indicate that the gut is 'hyperactive'. Loss of appetite is also possible and it is important that ME patients take heed of the advice in chapter 15 on nutrition if it continues too long.

Cardiac and Respiratory Problems

Palpitations: these can be a frightening symptom of ME and, accompanied by chest pains, often mark the onset of the illness. Shortness of breath is another worrying symptom but once again it usually occurs only at the start of the illness. When you have learnt to recognise the warning signs these attacks will become less frightening.

These are the major symptoms of ME and it is worth making the point that, unless these symptoms have been present for at least six months, it is unlikely that you have ME. Only a minority of people who go down with a viral infection go on to develop ME, so if you have some of these symptoms for only a short while, you probably won't get it.

Diagnosis of ME

Most doctors will make a diagnosis of ME on the clinical presentation of the symptoms. Many GPs now send their patients to be tested by Professor Mowbray, as if his test was conclusive proof as to whether they have ME. But as it is not a definitive test for ME it should not be used as diagnostic. (See Chapter 5.)

In many cases ME is a self-diagnosis by patients who realise what their disease is but cannot make their doctor accept it. In these cases the following questionnaire might be helpful. We have included it not as a means of self-diagnosis but so that you can record exactly what symptoms you are suffering. Some of the questions might not seem directly relevant to ME at first but they have been included to help you analyse your ME and your life in general. Answers to the questionnaire have been provided not as a hard diagnosis of ME, but are there to help explain some of the symptoms you might have.

The Questionnaire

Age:

Sex:

Occupation (if you have given up work when did you stop):

1. What is your present major symptom?

2. Do your symptoms fluctuate? Are they worse at any particular time of day? Of the month? Of the year?

3. How long have you had your symptoms?

4. Since your symptoms started, or in the last year, have had any of the following?

Headache (including migraine)
Catarrh

Mouth ulcers
Dyspepsia, abdominal distress, flatulence
Abdominal bloating
Pain in the stomach
Constipation
Diarrhoea
Variability of bowel function
Swelling of the throat or problems swallowing

Unusually slow or rapid heart beat
Palpitations
Pain in chest
Low blood pressure
High blood pressure

Feeling faint
Feeling unwell all over
Water retention

Bad dreams or very vivid dreams
Terrible thoughts on waking
Slow getting started in the morning
Insomnia
Difficulty waking up
Abrupt changes of state from well to unwell

Cramps in limbs
Aching muscles
Muscle twitching

Swollen, painful joints
Tingling all over
Sudden chills and tingling

Hypersensitivity to noise
Ringing in the ears
Giddiness
Nausea

Excessive sweating
Menstrual difficulties

'Dopey' feeling
Inability to think clearly
Irritability
Panic attacks
Feeling unreal, depersonalised
Lack of confidence
Mood swings
High mood (undue elation)
Low mood

General slowing down
General speeding up
Sudden tiredness after eating
Feeling totally drained and exhausted
'Flu like state that is not 'flu

5. Have you ever had asthma, hayfever, eczema, migraine, arthritis, colitis, depression or psychiatric illness?

6. Do you drink alcohol? If yes, what effect does it have on you?

7. Are you at present taking any drugs on prescription or any medication bought over the counter from your chemist?

8. What time do you get up?

9. What do you have for breakfast?

10. How many meals do you eat a day? At what times do you eat?

11. Do you normally have an after supper or late night snack?

12. If you normally eat regular meals what happens if you miss one or more meals?

13. When you are feeling rough do you ever eat something sweet and find that it makes you feel better quickly?

14. Do you now, or have you ever (say which), suffered from any of the following:
    (a) persistent fatigue not helped by rest?
    (b) over or underweight or history of fluctuating weight?
    (c) occasional swelling of the face, hands, abdomen or ankles?
    (d) palpitations, particularly after eating or coming on after eating?
    (e) excessive sweating, unrelated to exercise?

15. Since your symptoms started have you increased your intake of any foods or drinks (say which)?

16. Are there any foods or drinks you would feel deprived of it you could not have them? If so what are they?

17. Is there any food or drink you find yourself craving from time to time? When does the craving occur?

18. Are you on the Pill or have you ever taken it? If yes, when was this and for how long were you taking it?

19. Have you taken a course of antibiotics in the last three years? If yes, how many courses and when?

20. How many times a day do you have to sleep or lie down?

21. Do you take any exercise for pleasure? If yes, what and for how long?

22. Do you walk to work, or to catch a bus or train? How far do you have to walk?

23. Does exercise make you feel weak? How much exercise has this effect? How far can you walk before feeling tired?

24. Do you live alone?

25. If you live with someone, are they sympathetic to your health problems?

26. Do you have children? What age are they? Do they live at home?

27. How many hours a day are you able to relax totally?

28. What are your hobbies or favourite pursuits?

29. What is the level of stress in your life? Is the stress greater at home or at work?

30. Do you work or have you had to stop work because of your health? If yes, when?

31. If you work is your workplace noisy? If yes, is that from machines like typewriters or other people's conversations?

32. If you work, does your workplace smell?

33. If you work, are there machines in your workplace, for instance, photocopiers, VDUs?

34. Do you smoke? How many? Have you ever smoked? When did you give up?

35. If you do not smoke, do you live or work closely with people who do? Does the smoke affect you in any way?

36. How often, if at all, do you use household chemicals and toiletries like spray deodorants, hairsprays etc?

37. Do you heat your home or cook with gas, electricity or paraffin?

38. Do you have an acute nose (can you smell things when other people cannot)?

39. Are you aware of unpleasant reactions to chemicals?

40. Are there any chemical smells which you like (eg. petrol, paint, nail varnish)?

41. Have you ever been exposed to chemicals at work?

42. Does your condition improve if you are away from work? Or away from home? Or both?

43. Can you pinpoint the onset of your symptoms to one particular event in your life? What was it?

Answers to the Questionnaire

Questions 1–5. Symptoms.
Question 1. If you have ME you will have listed a wide range of symptoms. But the two major ones are extreme fatigue made worse by exercise, and what is often called brain fag, tremendous difficulty in thinking clearly and concentrating. Most doctors would not make a diagnosis of ME without these symptoms being present. In addition, coldness of the extremities is a good indicator of ME.

Question 2. Many ME sufferers notice that their symptoms fluctuate considerably. Women may find their symptoms exacerbated by pre-menstrual tension.

Question 3. No one should even start to consider that they might have ME unless their symptoms have been present for at least six months and the doctor has ruled out other causes. Many people experience a kind of post-viral fatigue syndrome after 'flu or another viral illness and this disappears within a few weeks or a few months at the most. And some viral infections, like glandular fever, will last this length of time anyway. Once you have had your symptoms for more than six months you should start thinking that a diagnosis of ME may be possible, although it is not always that clear cut.

Questions 4 and 5. Some of these questions relate to allergies. People with ME, and their close family, tend to have a history of allergies although nobody knows if this an important link or just a coincidence. What is known is that many ME sufferers have allergies. Sometimes it is not easy to recognise if you have an allergy so some of this questionnaire is designed to help you recognise if you have one. If you have ever suffered an atopic disease, like eczema or asthma, you are more likely to suffer allergies than other people.

Questions 6 and 7. Things that make ME worse.
Alcohol and medicines may make the symptoms of ME worse. Many ME sufferers report that if they have anything more than the equivalent of about one glass of wine their symptoms will be much worse the next day. Some find they get a hangover feeling on minute amounts of alcohol. Acetaldehyde is formed when alcohol is metabolised and this poison needs to be made safe in the liver. But it is quite likely that ME sufferers have livers that are not working 100 per cent efficiently so alcohol is not metabolised normally.

Some of the medicines prescribed by your doctor, or bought over the counter at the chemist, may make you feel worse, sometimes without you even realising it. If you have been used to taking antihistamines to relieve hayfever, for example, you may have forgotten that these drugs can make you very tired, adding to the tiredness of ME. If you are prescribed any drugs by your doctor or buy any from the chemist you should ask what side effects they have and if they are likely to make your ME symptoms worse. But do not stop taking a medicine that your doctor has prescribed without telling him or her why you are doing it. There may be nasty side effects from abruptly stopping medication so seek advice first.

Questions 8 to 17. Eating habits and food allergies.

Questions 8 to 13. If you miss out on breakfast or do not eat foods that will give you enough energy you could be setting yourself up for a day of excessive tiredness. Breakfast is one of the most important meals of the day. After several hours of not eating, your blood sugar will have dropped to very low levels. This hypoglycaemia, as it is known, can make you feel tired, irritable, weak, faint and dizzy, confused, weak and with an inability to concentrate.

You ought, therefore, to be getting every day off to a good start with a proper breakfast. That does not just mean a cup of coffee and piece of toast but a 'proper' breakfast with unrefined complex carbohydrates, protein and a little fat. Coffee will give you a temporary stimulus but after the initial effect you will feel worse than ever. Similarly, refined carbohydrates like white bread, croissants or sugary cereals will flood your system with an instant boost of sugar that will quickly be used up so you feel utterly deflated a couple of hours later. But foods with lots of protein, unrefined carbohydrates and a little fat will give your system a slow, steady rise in blood sugar that will be maintained at constant levels throughout the day. So you will not feel the sudden rushes of energy and troughs of fatigue and tiredness. The ideal breakfast would be a few rashers of bacon (grilled of course) or eggs or other protein and wholemeal toast: i.e. in spite of its cholesterol implications the good old English breakfast (see Chapter 12); or porridge or unsweetened muesli with banana.

Questions 14 to 17. These questions are all designed to help you recognise if you have a food allergy. The symptoms described in question 14 are all common food allergy symptoms. One of the surprising things about food allergies is that you will often crave the food that you have an allergy to. It is almost like an addiction. You feel subconsciously compelled to eat the food that gives you the allergy because you find it gives you a boost. Often it is this – the food that is most common in the diet – that is causing the allergy (see Chapter 7).

Questions 18 and 19. The Candida connection.
Overgrowth of the fungus *Candida albicans* may be a problem in ME sufferers as it is in many patients with an impaired immune system. The Pill and antibiotics alter the natural bacterial flora of the gut allowing other organisms to grow. One of the most troublesome of these is *Candida albicans* which can cause a range of symptoms including thrush, flatulence, abdominal pain, fatigue and irritability. If you have taken the Pill for a number of years or had more than one course of antibiotics within the last year you should suspect Candida (see Chapter 8) – especially if you have suffered from vaginitis or cystitis.

Questions 20 to 23. Sleep and exercise.
Most ME sufferers sleep more than normal people and at odd times of the day. But the amount of sleep you need is not so

important as whether that sleep is restful and refreshing. Waking up tired and exhausted means sleep is not performing its normal function of recovery. Some sufferers find their sleep pattern reversed so that they are awake at odd hours of the night and then sleep all day. There is no easy answer to this problem, and while not wishing to recommend unnecessary drugs, it is worth mentioning that some sufferers find sedative anti-depressants very helpful in restoring their sleep patterns to normal.

The inability to exercise without fatigue setting in quickly lies at the root cause of ME. If you record, every few months, how much exercise you are capable of you will have a good idea of how much you have or have not recovered.

Questions 24 to 31. Stress and the environment.
All these questions relate, in some way, to the level of stress in your life both at home and at work. It is impossible for us to give 'correct' answers to these questions. It is up to you to analyse whether you feel you have too much stress in your life. Obviously if your spouse or partner is unsympathetic to your health problems you will be under great pressure to improve and your relationship will be put under almost unbearable strain. That in itself can make you ill.

If you have had to give up work through ill health you may be under additional stress. (This is analysed in depth in chapter 10.)

Sometimes sitting down and thinking about the stresses in your life can help sort out ways through them. Alternatively you might like to contact other ME sufferers through an ME support group or ask your doctor to put you in touch with a stress counsellor or Relate (marriage guidance) counsellor.

Questions 32 to 42. Chemical and environmental allergies.
Like food allergies, chemical or environmental allergies may not be all that obvious. For instance, chemicals that you use every day at work or at home may just be part of your normal day-to-day life. You may not have even considered that using gas cookers may be causing some of your symptoms through giving off carbon monoxide gases and other chemicals. Or you may not have realised that the products you use to clean the house all give off powerful smells and chemicals that may be making your symptoms worse. Just as with food allergies, sometimes a particular chemical that you like the smell of, like nail varnish or petrol, may be the one that is causing your allergy. So look more closely around you and start asking 'Do I really need to use all

those chemicals'? Even if you are not allergic to chemicals, using fewer of them and not mixing them together can only be good for you, your family and your environment. If you answered yes to question 42 it is a very strong indication that chemical allergies are contributing to your ill health.

Question 43. Is it really ME?
You should think carefully about this question. Some sufferers can pinpoint the start of their ME to a specific event in their lives, and it may not just be a viral infection. While an acute viral illness is the starting point for some there are also those whose illness followed a major stressful event, for instance a bereavement, a divorce, changing jobs (even if you wanted the new job very badly), moving house, caring for a sick relative or having a baby. Any number of things could have happened before your illness that might have lowered your immune system and made you more receptive to a virus that turns into ME.

Even if your symptoms appeared gradually, if you analyse what happened in the months before your illness, you will very often find that you were stressed or undergoing more problems than normal. Just because you cannot attribute your ill health to a particular viral illness, or you find that maybe stress was the trigger for its onset, that does not make it any less of a disease.

The cause of your illness is not so important. What is important is coming to terms with having ME, setting yourself on the path to recovery and along the way dealing with those stresses that you may have been shoving under the carpet hoping they will go away. What is almost certain is that the stresses in your life will not go away on their own. You have to do something about them, and while it may be painful, it really will be the only way to clear your way for getting better.

5 What Causes ME?

A number of theories to explain ME have been put forward over the years. Probably the most plausible is that it is caused by a viral infection. There is evidence that the virus persists in the body to produce symptoms over many months or years, and there is also evidence that the viral infection damages the body's capacity to fight back and that it alters the immune system.

The Virus Theory
Much work has been done to find out if there is one specific virus that causes ME, but the current view is that any virus can cause it. Why some people do not recover from the infection when others sail through with just a few days illness is not clear. Are ME sufferers a special group of people who cannot combat viruses in the same way other people can? Are the viruses that cause ME a particularly 'nasty' strain that cause a more severe or more persistent infection than other strains?

At the moment we cannot answer all these questions, but from our knowledge of other viruses we do know that these theories are not too far-fetched. There are viruses that persist for many years, and there are also viruses with particularly virulent strains that cause more severe illnesses.

One of these is the Herpes virus. One type of Herpes virus causes cold sores that come back now and then, usually exacerbated by cold weather. People with cold sores do not have a new infection each time they have a cold sore. They carry the virus in their bodies all the time but it only shows as an infection at certain times, perhaps when the person is under a lot of stress at work or during particularly cold weather. Perhaps whatever virus it is that causes ME has somehow taken on the characteristics of the Herpes virus and manages to persist in the body for many months or years.

From our knowledge of the influenza viruses we know that different strains evolve every year so there is always a new type of 'flu that we will not be immune to. However, when there is a 'flu epidemic not everyone catches the new type of 'flu – their immune systems may be equipped to deal with it. Why they should be able to combat a new strain of 'flu while others fall like flies is not clear – perhaps the same mechanism is at work in ME.

Before we ponder why some sufferers might be more prone to viral infection it is important to have some basic understanding of how viruses infect the body.

There are many thousands of viruses that infect humans, animals, birds, insects and even plants. Many common diseases are caused by viruses, for instance, influenza, measles, mumps, chicken pox and the common cold. But viruses that cause the same diseases may not be the same from country to country or even from one town to another. Different strains of viruses may develop in a fairly small area and that may explain why a family that moves from one town to another, in a different part of the country, may suffer more colds or bouts of 'flu than normal in the first few months they are there.

It is not entirely understood why different strains of viruses develop. But in the case of the influenza virus it is thought that animals might act as mixing vessels so that viruses from humans and, for instance, poultry might combine in another animal to produce a totally different strain of the virus.

Humans can become infected with viruses in many different ways. The most common is just by breathing them in. Someone with a cold will release virus-contaminated droplets every time they sneeze or cough or even just speak normally. These droplets will be breathed in through other people's noses or mouths and the virus passed on. Just shaking hands with someone who has a cold can pass the virus on if you do not wash your hands again before touching your own nose or mouth. Kissing someone with influenza can also be an effective way of catching a virus, as can sharing a towel.

Some viruses multiply in the gastrointestinal tract and can easily be passed on through poor sanitation or even at swimming pools. Viruses like poliomyelitis or hepatitis-A are good examples of viruses that multiply in the gut. In countries with poor sanitation, viruses in the faeces may contaminate supplies of drinking water and cause widespread infection. Even in well-developed countries infected faeces that are discharged into sea-water may contaminate shellfish which will infect whoever eats them if they are not cooked properly.

Large amounts of viruses can be excreted in the faeces and it is essential that anyone who handles food washes their hands after using the toilet. Many cases of infection would be avoided if this simple rule was strictly adhered to.

The skin is another barrier that can be crossed by viruses. In the case of cold sores, viruses may be present in the sores themselves and can easily be transmitted through small cuts in the skin of another person. And, of course, everyone must by now be aware of the dangers of transmitting viruses through blood-to-blood contact with other people. Since the AIDS epidemic began drug addicts have been exhorted not to share needles with other drug addicts for the very real danger of transmitting not just AIDS but other highly infectious diseases like hepatitis-B.

Although there are many ways a virus can enter the body, just having a virus does not mean that you will automatically go down with an infection. If only very small amounts of virus have been transmitted you are unlikely to succumb to an infection because your immune system will quickly wipe it out.

Often you will already be immune to the virus that has invaded your body. Perhaps you have already had a bout of the same 'flu strain earlier in the year and have developed antibodies against it. But if you have not been infected with a particular virus before you will be susceptible. There are many hundreds of viruses that cause the common cold so if you have spent all winter with cold after cold you can be certain it was not the same virus that was causing the infection each time. While it is possible for us to have many colds throughout our life, we generally only get one attack of measles or chickenpox or mumps. That is because after one infection we develop a natural immunity to the disease.

It is also possible to acquire an 'artificial' immunity to a disease through vaccination. While most people remember childhood bouts of measles as nothing more than very irritating illnesses that went away within a week, for some people these 'mild' diseases can maim or even kill. So small amounts of live or 'killed' vaccine given as an injection, or in the case of polio as a liquid that you swallow, enable your body to build up immunity without you contracting the disease.

Once inside the human body viruses multiply rapidly. But they can only multiply within living cells because they need to use some of the genetic ingredients found in every living cell to reproduce. These genetic ingredients are the DNA that is the code for every chemical reaction that occurs in the body. The codes for every single enzyme produced to make our bodies work properly are found in the genetic material of each cell. So it is not surprising that when this genetic material is 'hijacked' by viruses for their own means we suffer the symptoms of influenza, or measles, or chickenpox.

When viruses get into the body the first thing they do is latch onto the surface of cells with special receptors. The virus then releases all its contents into the cell. It uses the RNA in the cell to make copies of its own genetic material to produce 'daughter' viruses which are then released to go and infect other cells. When enough 'daughter' viruses have been produced we suffer the symptoms of the illness. The incubation period is the time that elapses between the virus getting into the body and producing symptoms. Different viruses attack cells in different parts of the body. For instance, in measles and chickenpox the virus attacks the skin cells, while in the common cold it is the nasal cavity and the throat cells that are most affected. The viruses that produce symptoms are called virulent but there are some viruses that do not cause symptoms and these are called asymptomatic.

During the acute stage of a viral infection it is usually fairly easy for the doctor to make a diagnosis. The symptoms of the infection are usually unique to each virus and if there is a viral infection 'going around' the doctor is likely to have seen many other cases.

In the acute stage of the illness it is possible to grow cultures of the virus in the microbiologist's laboratory. If the doctor is not sure which virus is causing a disease it is normal to take a swab of the affected area, for instance the nose or throat. The swab will contain cells contaminated with the virus. When these cells are grown in the laboratory the characteristic pattern of growth for each virus tells the microbiologist which one is present. But later on in the infection it might not be possible to culture the virus so a diagnosis may be made from blood tests that show changes in the blood in response to an infection.

One of the most obvious changes in the blood of someone infected with a virus is that antibodies to a particular virus will be produced by the lymphocytes – white blood cells that are particularly active against viral infections. Other changes in the blood can also indicate that the patient is fighting an infection, changes in the ratio of white blood cells and red blood cells, changes in the types of white blood cells that are present. Different white cells fight different types of infection, for instance, some work against bacteria and parasites, while others work specifically against viruses.

That is the acute stage of the illness. What happens in a prolonged viral infection such as ME is not clear-cut. Sometimes in an illness that has lasted many months, the symptoms may be caused by the after effects of the virus and not by a continuing infection with the virus. For instance, sometimes the common cold virus can damage nerve endings in the head and neck which causes pain for many months or even years afterwards.

Doctors find it virtually impossible to diagnose ME with any of the methods used for acute illness because none of the standard tests work. Viruses can rarely be cultured after the acute stage of the illness, and this is not surprising as ME is probably not caused by a continuing acute infection but by the after affects of viral infection.

However there are reports in medical literature of isolation of viruses and viral antigens (proteins that make up the viral wall) from people with ME. In the three Scottish outbreaks mentioned in Chapter 3 antibodies to a group of viruses were cultured from patients with ME. Reporting in the *Journal of Infection* in 1985 Dr Peter Behan, Dr Wilhelmina Behan and Dr Eleanor Bell described their studies of 50 patients with the same primary symptom: 'gross fatigue made worse by exercise' and all reported a virus or viral-like illness as the initial event in their disease.

Not only did these researchers identify muscle disorders in these patients but they found raised levels of antibodies to Coxsackie B viruses. 35 of the 50 patients had raised levels of antibodies to Coxsackie B virus – that is 70 per cent of the patients. When one of the researchers conducted random tests in the general population only four per cent had raised antibody levels to Coxsackie B virus.

In addition, 70 per cent of the patients had an impaired T-cell function, that is some of the white blood cells designed to fight viral infections were missing. This depletion of T-cells is seen in other viral illnesses. The patients also showed immune disorders similar to those seen in multiple sclerosis and in auto-immune disorders such as systemic *Lupus erythematosus* and in the immune disorders seen in those who have received kidney or other organ transplants.

There are several types of T-cells but two of the most important are the T-helper and the T-suppressor cells. The researchers measured the ratios of these cells to get some idea of the immune status of the patients. They found very depleted ratios of these cells similar to the ratios seen in patients with AIDS, the ultimate immune deficiency disease. However, ME is not AIDS. AIDS is characterised by swollen glands all over the body, opportunistic infections and dementia which are totally different symptoms to ME. AIDS is usually fatal while, to date, no one has actually died from ME. And there is a specific blood test for AIDS that identifies antibodies to human immunodeficiency virus – this is not the virus that causes ME. But research into the effect of AIDS on the immune system could one day be very helpful in the research into ME as more is understood about the immune system and how it works. While Behan, Behan and Bell's work showed clearly that the Coxsackie-B viruses were implicated in the outbreaks of ME in Scotland in the early 1980s there is work to show that other viruses belonging to the same group may also cause ME.

Coxsackie-B viruses are part of a group of viruses called the enteroviruses. There are around 70 enteroviruses altogether and the Coxsackie-B viruses are just six of them. According to Professor James Mowbray, Professor of Immunopathology at London's St Mary's Hospital, any of the enteroviruses could potentially cause ME. Professor Mowbray has worked with ME patients for many years and had long harboured the suspicion that the enteroviruses were to blame, but it was not until January 1988 that he was able to publish work that gave definite proof.

In *The Lancet* of 23 January 1988, Professor Mowbray and six colleagues described how they had found evidence of persistent infection with enteroviruses in many of their patients. Using a highly specific blood test they found that 51 per cent of a group of 87 ME patients had enterovirus antigens in their blood, that is, particles of enterovirus proteins were present in the blood. When they tested the blood of normal people they could find no evidence of enterovirus antigens. When the positive patients were tested four months later 89 per cent were still positive.

Professor Mowbray also tried to isolate enteroviruses from the faeces of a group of patients – which is the standard way to get material for viral culture of enteroviruses – but the success for this was more limited. He isolated enteroviruses from the faeces of 22 per cent of the patients and said that the results were probably less conclusive because antibodies in the gut tend to neutralise the virus. The blood test was obviously a more effective test for detecting the enterovirus antigens, as well as being more pleasant for both patients and doctor.

Professor Mowbray tested a number of the patients a year later and found that considerable numbers still had the enterovirus antigens in their blood. His test is now often regarded by doctors as a test for ME, but as Mowbray is only too ready to admit himself, it is not a foolproof test as only half the patients show a positive response.

'It approximates to a screening process,' he says. 'But it's not a test for ME, it's a diagnostic test for some of the conditions that might lead to ME.'

So while the enteroviruses might cause ME in a large majority of people there are still some who have ME but not a positive test. Where do these people fit in? To find out we have to go back to Dr Melvin Ramsay, one of the founding fathers of ME research.

'It would seem likely that any virus may "trigger" the disease if the immunological state of the person is defective,' he says in his book *Postviral Fatigue Syndrome: The Saga of Royal Free Disease*.

It may be that enteroviruses are a major trigger of ME but not the only group of viruses capable of acting as a trigger. In the USA, infections of the Epstein Barr virus have been known to cause outbreaks of prolonged and atypical illnesses that are virtually indistinguishable from ME. Yet the Epstein Barr virus is a member of the Herpes family of viruses and is typically associated with infectious mononucleosis, an illness that is very similar to glandular fever. There has been some doubt whether infectious mononucleosis could persist to produce the long-term symptoms seen in ME patients. But since 1984 there has been a growing body of research using modern viral culture techniques that prove that the Epstein Barr virus can persist for many months or years. Epstein Barr virus is massively under-recognised. However, around 80 per cent of people have been exposed to it by the time they reach adolescence. It is well known that the Herpes viruses have a tendency to reactivate so it would hardly be surprising if this virus caused persistent infection with relapses.

ME may not only be caused by persistent infection with a virus but the viral infection may actually damage the body's tissues and metabolism so that it does not function properly or may take many years to recover. Or the virus may only persist in people with a defective immune system or it may actually damage the immune system of susceptible people. It is now known from studies of the AIDS virus that there are viruses capable of damaging the immune system, and Behan, Behan and Bell's work in Glasgow suggests that the Coxsackie-B virus may hinder the immune system so it is incapable of fighting the virus in the normal way. All these questions will only be answered with more research.

Who Gets ME?
In the UK there are probably close to 200,000 people with ME although it is difficult to give a true figure. The huge response to Sue Finlay's article in *The Observer* and the greater awareness of the illness among the general public have produced an ever increasing number of people who think that maybe they have ME.

ME has been nicknamed Yuppie 'Flu by the popular press because in the USA it was originally thought that it affected mostly young, successful professionals in their twenties. But it is not exclusively a Yuppie disease. Dr Paul Cheney, a family doctor in Incline, Nevada, where there was an outbreak that affected at least 200 of his patients says: 'I don't think this virus can distinguish whether you are a Yuppie or not. Yuppies get the diagnosis because they have the wherewithal to stand up to physicians and say, "You are wrong – I'm not crazy." Only people from higher socio-economic groups, and highly educated people, have the ability to get through the roadblocks that exist to this diagnosis. It requires persistence and the ability to challenge medical authority.'

Professor Anthony Komaroff, Professor of Medicine at Harvard University agrees that ME does not hit only Yuppies: 'Well educated, high achievers would be the least likely to take no for an answer. But in our experience we are seeing people from all walks of life, lots of non-Yuppies, blue collar workers, blacks and whites.' And in Britain, when the ME Action Campaign sent out questionnaires in April 1988, only 14 per cent of respondents were in their twenties. 27 per cent were in their thirties, 23 per cent in the forties and 20 per cent in their fifties.

Some of the outbreaks have occurred among communities of women and, for a long time, it was believed that women were more prone to ME. Research by the two ME charities shows that women sufferers do seem to outnumber men by at least two to one, but it is not solely a woman's disease as the outbreaks among the Swiss Army battalions show. It may be that men are reticent about admitting to this type of illness and with publicity more may be encouraged to seek help. Another factor is that women suffer more from the symptoms of Candida than men (see Chapter 8) and these symptoms can easily be confused with ME.

People in the health care professions also seem to suffer more than other groups of people. Why this should be is a mystery. It may be that these groups have more contact with different viruses than other groups of people so they have more chance of catching a viral infection and thereby contracting ME. Or it may be that they are more concerned with getting a diagnosis and are more forceful in their efforts to find a name for their unexplained and persistent ill health. Or it may be that they are more likely to go on working when they are already under considerable stress and therefore do not take the rest necessary to stave off ME in its early stages.

Is ME Catching?

Viruses can be passed from person-to-person as we discussed earlier on in this chapter, but they are normally transmitted during the initial stages of the disease when the virus first gets into the body. That does not mean the person getting the virus will necessarily develop ME, he or she might just be ill for a few days. So a virus may be passed from person-to-person but, in general, ME is not.

There have been cases of people in the same family contracting ME. For instance, in the outbreak in West Kilbride a 41-year-old airline steward contracted ME and then a few weeks later his eight-year-old daughter went down with an identical illness. Both of them had similar levels of Coxsackie-B virus antibodies. It is rare that members of the same family go down with ME, and although the whole family may suffer from the initial infection, they would not normally all contract ME.

Although the virus is thought to persist within the body of the ME sufferer it is probably deep within the body, for instance, in the muscles or in the heart, or the intestine and not in the respiratory tract where it would be more likely to be easily transmitted. And although ME sufferers make a poor immune response to the virus they probably neutralise it with neutralising antibodies so that it cannot be passed on.

As in any virus infection, the person who is sick will be infectious in the first few days but after that is probably not.

However anyone who suffers a viral infection should take precautions not to pass it on – by covering the mouth when sneezing, washing hands regularly and not touching the nose and mouth. Until more is known about ME it may be advisable for people with the disease not to become blood donors.

The Hyperventilation Theory
On 17 July 1988 the front page headline in *The Sunday Times* was 'Yuppie flu is all in the mind, say doctors'. Researchers from London's Charing Cross Hospital told *The Sunday Times* medical correspondent that they thought ME was nothing more than tiredness brought on by striving to achieve unattainable ambitions.

They said the problems in ME patients of fatigue, loss of memory, sleep disturbances, headaches, nausea, bowel upsets, and loss of concentration were identical to those seen in heart patients. However, the symptoms were not caused by heart problems or a viral infection but simply by overbreathing or hyperventilation. The Charing Cross team had carefully selected 20 ME patients and found hyperventilation in all of them, although Ramsay and Scott said they had not found over-breathing in the 500 patients they saw (Chapter 3).

While this sounds ludicrous to anyone who suffers from ME, the theory behind it is not. Hyperventilation is a very common problem – it is estimated that around half the people visiting doctors' surgeries are overbreathing. Yet rarely are they advised to breathe properly and, in fact, the problem is barely recognised and they are merely handed a prescription for their anxiety, or insomnia or even angina.

To understand how hyperventilation may affect the physiology of the body it is important to understand the mechanism of breathing. Our bodies have two ways of breathing, one using the chest (thoracic breathing) and one using the abdomen (diaphragmatic breathing). Abdominal breathing is the most efficient breathing mechanism. By taking in eight to 12 breaths a minute using your diaphragm, you can take in as much air as you can in the 14 to 18 breaths a minute you would take using your chest. Over weeks, months and years abdominal breathing is the most energy efficient and it is the body's normal way of taking in oxygen and exchanging it with carbon dioxide.

Chest breathing is an emergency mechanism. It is the breathing you would use to get oxygen into the lungs quickly in order to run for the bus or take some exercise. It probably evolved as an emergency mechanism to give the body enough oxygen to run away from danger fast, but if you continue to chest breathe after the emergency is over your body will not only take in too much oxygen, it will lose too much carbon dioxide. While carbon dioxide is generally thought of as a waste product it is important in many of the body's chemical processes. A drop in carbon dioxide in the blood can change the acidity of the blood dramatically. The blood becomes more alkaline and this causes the arteries to constrict, cutting the blood supply to vital organs like the brain, liver, kidneys, muscles etc.

In only four minutes of hyperventilating the blood supply to the brain can be cut by half, making you dizzy, unable to think straight, or feel faint. The increase in blood alkalinity also affects the mechanism of calcium exchange between the blood and nerves and muscles which results in the symptoms of tingling, numbness, trembling, chest tightness.

Many physical symptoms such as panic attacks, angina, chronic fatigue, migraine, even heart disease have been attributed to hyperventilation. According to Dr Peter Nixon, senior consultant cardiologist at the Charing Cross Hospital, there are no heart patients who do not overbreathe. For several years he has organised a relaxation programme for his patients to help them to get over the problem and put the chemical processes right. Many of his patients have been greatly helped, and Dr Nixon now believes that hyperventilation could be as important as other risk factors for heart disease like smoking, high blood pressure and eating a high cholesterol diet.

Why do people start to hyperventilate? Any situation where there is a sense of loss of control can precipitate hyper-ventilation, for instance going for an important job interview. Or a woman worrying, when her husband is late home from the office every night, that he is having an affair. Or the man who suddenly discovers that his wife is capable of leading her own independent life and who might not need him anymore. Some stress researchers believe that people find it easier to deal with hyperventilation-induced illness than the real stresses and strains of their life. People feel they can cope with angina or migrainous headaches but are afraid to face up to their own emotions. They unknowingly hide behind hyperventilation. But they do not realise they are doing it because the link between a real physical disease and bad breathing can be very obscure.

Hyperventilation is very difficult to detect. Despite its prevalence there are not millions of people walking the street puffing and panting all day. It can be so unobtrusive that trained doctors can fail to find it.

Finding that hyperventilation was a big problem in their clients, researchers from The Stress Research Unit at London's St Bartholomew's Hospital developed a small carbon dioxide monitor (about the size of a matchbox) that can be clamped to the body. It takes measurements through the skin of the levels of carbon dioxide in the blood and can given a graphic account to doctors and patients of how much of their problems are a result of hyperventilation.

So can ME be caused by hyperventilating? At the moment it is impossible to give a definite answer. At the time of the *Sunday Times* article Dr Nixon had treated only 20 ME patients at his clinic for hyperventilation, just a tiny proportion of the estimated 200,000 people who are thought to have ME. While he claims to have cured some of the patients completely, others are not totally cured by being taught to breathe properly and confront their stresses. Learning how to breathe properly could help some people reduce their symptoms but if ME is caused by a persistent viral infection it is not going to get rid of the virus and the real symptoms of ME. A proportion of patients who have had ME for some time may have a disordered breathing system. Dr Len McEwen who has treated many ME patients, says overbreathing may be learned as a response to the physical weakness and anxiety which are major symptoms of ME. Learning how to breathe properly could help many people reduce these symptoms (see Chapter 12) but it is most unlikely to completely cure them.

6 What Makes ME Worse?

Every ME sufferer will come to recognise situations or activities that make their particular set of symptoms worse, but there are some things that affect everyone and can even set back the course of recovery. So it is important for all sufferers to be aware of what they can and cannot do, although every person will be different and it is impossible to set strict guidelines to follow. While one person might be reduced to a heap of quivering jelly after a short walk to the shops, another might get away with nothing more than an evening of mild fatigue. Every sufferer must learn to recognise their own limitations and be guided by them.

Exercise

For many sufferers, ME comes during their most active years. It has been suggested that because ME tends to affect people who are in general more active and energetic than their counterparts, they notice the change in their activity levels more. Certainly someone who went running every day and played squash twice a week would notice fatigue more than a person who sat in front of the television night after night.

Many very active people equate exercise with keeping fit. So when they become ill with ME they feel they should exercise more to get fit again. But that is the worst thing anyone with ME can do. At the moment we are experiencing a fitness boom and everyone is told that exercise is good for them. So it is frustrating to have an illness where exercise is positively bad for you.

Severe fatigue and tiredness are the commonest symptoms experienced by people with ME after a bout of exercise. This fatigue is very difficult to describe to non-sufferers. Some people feel they are completely drained of energy, like a battery that needs recharging. Others feel so weak and tired that even the effort of lifting a cup of tea is too much to cope with.

A 39-year-old male company director said: 'I have always been a strong, swift walker and a few years ago I completed a 50-mile walk in one day. Even though I had lost the fitness for that, I could still walk long distances easily, but after Christmas 1984 a walk, or should I say a stroll, of only 100 yards or so would leave me sitting on a wall or a tree stump, gasping for air – a total wreck.'

Why is ME affected by exercise? Although there is no clear-cut answer a clue might be found in the way the virus affects the muscles. A number of studies have observed that the muscles of ME sufferers are abnormal – there are changes in the contents of the muscle cells and some key cellular enzymes appear to be missing. Work done with a technique called nuclear magnetic resonance has revealed that the muscle metabolism does not follow the normal pathways. This means lactic acid, a waste product formed during exercise, builds up in the muscle cells.

During exercise the muscles of the ME patient seem to switch to a different metabolic pathway from that which a normal person's muscles would take, so that the glycogen, the substance that gives the muscle energy to work, is broken down too early. Lactic acid is produced as a result of this breakdown of glycogen but, because it is produced so early in the process, the next steps in the pathway are not ready to get rid of it, so it accumulates in the muscles.

When lactic acid builds up in the muscles it changes the alkalinity of the muscle cells and of the blood flowing in and around the muscles. This means that the chemical reactions needed to keep the muscles going, cannot occur because they do not have the right conditions. In addition to producing lactic acid too early, ME sufferers do not seem able to get rid of this waste product as quickly as normal people and this may account for the time it takes an ME sufferer to recover from exercise.

In his observations of ME sufferers, Dr Melvin Ramsay said it took some patients three to four days to recover from moderate exercise, like walking half-a-mile, while it might take two or three weeks to recover from more strenuous exercise. If it takes up to three weeks to recover from doing exercise this means that lactic acid is staying in the muscles for a long period of time and there is no knowing what damage this abnormal acidity might cause. So the advice most doctors would give to ME patients is to rest, particularly in the early stages of the disease, in order to avoid further damage to the muscles.

'Absolute rest in the early stages of the disease can prove a very strong determining factor in the outcome,' said Dr Ramsay. 'Relapses resulting from excessive physical and/or mental stress or after a further virus infection are an accepted feature of the disease.'

A graphic example of the way exercise can affect the process of recovery was given by a 36-year-old patient called Jill. She described how she was gradually recovering from ten years of suffering with ME and had taken on part-time voluntary work with a local youth club:

'By about May 1985 I was virtually normal again. Then one night my youth hockey team were one short and I stepped in. Within half-an-hour, all my old symptoms were back in force and by the end of the evening it was as if I had gone back ten years.

'I spent the next year making very little progress and I'm now gradually recovering again, although I'm very prone to setbacks at any hint of stress. I'm now back to the stage where I can't carry a shopping bag without spending the evening in some discomfort with trembling muscles and aches and pains. I had totally forgotten that ME could get me this way.'

It is very easy for doctors to tell patients to rest but for people who have been used to doing lots of exercise and living an energetic life this can be very difficult. Many sufferers will remember times when they were well and exercise gave them a feeling of elation, bursting energy and a zest for life. It hardly seems possible that exercise can do harm.

What every ME sufferer has to recognise is that he or she is ill. ME is not an obvious physical disability in the way that a broken leg is, and it is all too easy for sufferers, their friends and their families to forget they are really ill. But no one would contemplate jogging round the park with a broken leg and the same should be true of ME.

Exercise is not the way to get back to full health because the muscles are not functioning normally. But after six months or so of absolute rest most sufferers will be itching to do some sort of activity. It would be wrong to ban all exercise after six months because many patients have found that they can cope with very moderate exercise and it helps to tone up the muscles that have become wasted through months of inactivity. The trick is to take it very slowly and not to overdo things.

Every ME sufferer has to learn their own limitations. Many patients find that a ten-minute walk or a five-minute swim will not result in symptoms, but a 15-minute walk or a ten-minute swim might. It is important to stop doing the exercise before any symptoms start to appear and not force yourself to the very limits.

With an illness like ME even six months of rest will not return you to your former capacity. If you regularly jogged five miles a night before your illness it may be that you will only be able to walk 100 yards up the road afterwards. If you try and do what you were capable of before, the result will be a predictable several days of fatigue, malaise and other symptoms exacerbated by exercise.

The type of exercise you do, once you feel you are capable, is just as important as how long you do it for. The best things are probably slow walking and swimming. Generally, any exercise where you can control the pace yourself and the time you spend doing it is the best, as then you can stop when you want to. Team games are probably the worst because you will be constantly on the go and have to produce unpredictable bursts of energy, and you will not be able to stop and rest when you want to. Any strenuous sport like squash or rowing is unsuitable for the person trying to recover from ME.

Eventually you will learn what activities you are capable of and how long you will be able to do them. If you do feel like exerting yourself, then you must realise that you will probably spend the next few days or even weeks recovering. So listen to what your body is telling you.

Tea, Coffee, Alcohol
Tea and coffee are amongst the most popular drinks consumed in the UK and there can be few people who do not start the day with a pot of tea or a mug of coffee. But these drinks are not popular just for their taste, they contain the chemical caffeine which we use, probably without realising it, for its stimulant effects. If your energy is flagging during a shopping trip do you pop to the local café for a cup of tea? Do you feel you cannot start the day without a cup of coffee? You are relying on caffeine as a 'pick-me-up', a stimulant to keep you going. There is nothing wrong with this as long as you are healthy and your need for such a stimulus does not control you – you need to control it.

In the case of caffeine, the word stimulant does not just mean giving you get up and go. As a stimulant there is hardly any part of the body or chemical reaction in the body that is not affected by caffeine. It should really be considered a drug rather than a harmless constituent of tea or coffee, and if you are trying to recover from a disease such as ME you need to know what effect drugs like caffeine are having on your body. In some cases caffeine and similar stimulants can make your ME symptoms worse and this will prevent recovery.

The average cup of tea contains around 50 milligrams of caffeine, while a cup of coffee will have about 100 milligrams. Pharmacological effects can be seen with anything from 50 milligrams upwards so you should take your breakfast cuppa very seriously. Caffeine is absorbed very quickly into the body and within ten minutes of drinking a cup of coffee you will notice its effects and they may last for several hours.

The first thing caffeine does is stimulate parts of the brain that are responsible for thought, controlling the heart rate, respiration and muscular coordination. It will raise your metabolic rate so that you burn off more calories and it triggers the production of the hormone insulin. It also stimulates the heart rate, making your heart beat faster. It relaxes the muscles of the digestive system and also has a diuretic effect on the body increasing the volume of urine you excrete.

Hypoglycaemia
If you suffer from palpitations, bowel or bladder problems you would be wise to avoid caffeine drinks as they will exacerbate any symptoms you might have. But one of the most serious side-effects of drinking caffeine is its effects on your blood sugar levels. Many ME sufferers have hypoglycaemia or low blood suger. (There are three types of hypoglycaemia. Severe hypo-glycaemia is caused by a disease such as cancer in which tumours of the pancreas or liver produce insulin. Diabetic hypoglycaemia occurs when a diabetic who takes insulin takes too much, resulting in a rapid decrease in blood glucose levels. Reactive hypoglycaemia, the type often experienced by ME sufferers, means low blood sugar caused by metabolic problems.)

A person is hypoglycaemic when levels of blood glucose fall too low, producing a range of symptoms including weakness, faintness, anxiety, cold sweats, irritability, hunger, mood swings, headaches and a rapid heart rate. It is caused when too much insulin is produced from the pancreas. Insulin is the hormone that takes glucose out of the blood and transports it to cells where it is used for energy or stored. When a lot of insulin is produced it rapidly lowers the blood sugar. This is not so important for the muscles, but the brain needs a constant flow of blood with the right level of glucose, so it is no surprise that many of the symptoms arising from low blood sugar occur in the brain.

Caffeine consumption is a common cause of hypoglycaemia because it produces a rapid rise in insulin that quickly lowers blood sugar. If you drink a cup of coffee on its own first thing in the morning you are heading for trouble. Your blood sugar level will already be low from your overnight fast and drinking coffee or tea will lower it still further, leading to hypoglycaemia about mid-morning.

Hypoglycaemia will make you feel hungry and produce a great temptation to snack on sweet sugary foods. When you eat sugary foods you are perpetuating your hypoglycaemia; sugar stimulates excessive production of insulin and lowers your blood sugar still further. If you eat a meal that takes longer to digest, for instance a chicken sandwich made with wholewheat bread, you will not get the rush of insulin production that causes all these problems. If you have hypoglycaemic episodes you should avoid tea, coffee, colas and other fizzy drinks with caffeine added and try eating four or five small meals a day of unrefined carboyhydrates and protein. This type of meal takes longer to digest so there is a steady rise in insulin rather than a rush.

Alcohol
For similar reasons you should avoid alcoholic drinks. Alcohol is really just a refined carbohydrate, like white sugar, and it stimulates the rush of insulin production, leading to hypoglycaemia. Alcohol also has many adverse effects on the body. One of the most important of these as far as ME sufferers are concerned is that it depletes almost every vitamin and many of the minerals that we eat or store in our body. If you have ME you probably also have higher requirements for vitamins and minerals. Not only do you need more to fight this illness but your absorption of these nutrients may be impaired.

A more sinister aspect of alcohol for people with ME is the effect it has on the liver. Many sufferers report that just one glass of wine will make them extremely sleepy, sometimes within half-an-hour after drinking. Or they spend the next day feeling excessively hungover after drinking only a small amount. All this points to some sort of defect in the liver where 95 per cent of the alcohol is metabolised. One of the steps along the pathway to producing energy from alcohol is the production of acetaldehyde, a potent toxin. If this is allowed to linger in the body it could give rise to many of the symptoms that ME sufferers describe. It may be that the metabolic pathway converting alcohol to energy is disrupted in some way, allowing this poison to accumulate. For this reason it would be wise to avoid alcohol as the long-term effects of acetaldehyde lingering in the body are not fully understood.

Most of those few people who have made a substantial recovery from ME have had the good sense to cut out tea, coffee and alcohol. Angela feels a lot better since she has drastically reduced her tea drinking. Hilary McLennan says 'Now I have cut them out, one little sip gives me such a buzz.' It is interesting to watch people at social gatherings and see how talkative and energetic they become when the caffeine or alcohol first gets into their system. Then the effect begins to wear off, their blood sugar drops and you can see them begin to droop and go quieter and quieter. They become very much in need of another 'fix'.

Robert, who has been to many meetings of ME Support groups, has noticed the same thing. 'Many of the sufferers arrive looking more than a bit downcast and under the weather, the journey has obviously tired them out. Most of them have a cup of tea and at once they start chatting away nineteen-to-the-dozen. But about an hour to an hour-and-a-half later, the conversation begins to die away and everyone starts to wilt. Some go very silent, others start saying how much their energy levels go up and down and how they tire so easily now they have got ME.'

Of course, people with ME get tired. Fatigue is the hallmark of the illness. But if all sufferers watched their caffeine consumption and ate only complex rather than simple carbohydrates (more on this in Chapter 15) their energy levels would be much more constant and not be subject to the ups and downs that, for many, are so bewildering. Fluctuating energy levels are reported by almost all sufferers and fluctuating energy levels produce mood swings. The displays of irritability and feelings of depression that are often part of ME can be kept much more under control by careful attention to diet.

7 The Allergy Connection

It might seem strange that a book about ME should devote a whole chapter to allergies. After all, you might say, ME is a viral illness and surely has nothing to do with having allergies? Well, yes and no. Yes, most cases of ME are probably caused by a virus but there are many other things that may be contributing to your ill health and food and chemical allergies are among the most important and least recognised.

It seems that when patients contract ME their immune systems go awry and one of the results of this is an increased susceptibility to allergies. These are not the typical everyday allergies you might associate easily with particular foods but a more sinister form of 'masked' or hidden allergy that cannot be so readily diagnosed.

Every one knows of the immediate allergic reaction that occurs in people who suffer from hayfever. When they become exposed to pollen they start sneezing, their eyes water and their noses run, they often start wheezing and coughing. Similarly, you might know someone who reacts to strawberries or shellfish and cannot eat either of those foods without developing a severe rash or swollen mouth. They avoid these allergic reactions by simply avoiding those foods. The cause and effect in these allergic reactions is so obvious that the cause is avoided.

The types of allergies you may not have come across are those called food intolerance or chemical sensitivities. These have a more insidious onset and can be responsible for a wide range of symptoms without you even realising where they spring from. Symptoms caused by food and chemical intolerances include fatigue, headaches, depression, anxiety, bowel upsets, swollen abdomen, chest pains and palpitations, difficulty with breathing, aching or painful muscles and painful joints.

Many of these symptoms are identical to those caused by ME. So if you think you have ME, but are not sure, one of the first things you should do is check whether some, or all, of your symptoms are caused by allergies. We are not saying that if you have ME you will necessarily get 100 per cent better by tracking down your allergies and dealing with them, but we suspect that eliminating problem foods and cutting down on exposure to chemicals will do a lot to alleviate your symptoms. Some patients who have followed this course of action have discovered that all their symptoms were caused by allergies and they have managed to discard the label of ME sufferer.

Food Allergies and How to Test for Them
It is important to understand that you may be suffering from an allergy without even realising it. If you have completed the questionnaire in Chapter 4 you will already have some idea of whether you have a food or chemical allergy. If you have not completed the questionnaire you might find it helpful to do so now before reading any further. If the answers to some of the questions do not make sense at the moment, they may do so after you have read this chapter.

Wheat, dairy products and eggs are the commonest foods causing allergies in Britain. Indeed most food allergies are caused by foods that we eat every day, often several times a day. Why is this?

It has been found that many people with food intolerances are unconsciously 'addicted' to the very foods and drinks that cause the reaction – rather like a junkie is addicted to drugs. If you stop eating the food that is at the root of your allergy you will experience withdrawal symptoms in the form of headache, fatigue and malaise. So, subconsciously, you make sure you eat that food every day, keeping yourself on a maintenance dose so that you do not have to experience those symptoms again. For instance, if you are allergic to wheat and wheat products you might start the day off with a couple of slices of toast, have biscuits with your cup of coffee later in the morning, and a sandwich for lunch, pasta for your evening meal and perhaps a late-night snack of cheese on toast. Since it takes on average four days for food to make its way through the digestive system you are unlikely ever to be completely free of the allergenic food if it is very common in your diet. Your body will adapt by not producing an immediate severe allergic reaction, but instead you will suffer from a wide range of symptoms that, at first sight, do not seem related to food allergy.

You may not realise the connection but you may be experiencing the same ups and downs that an addict suffers when taking drugs or being deprived of them. By eating the food you are allergic to you may experience a 'high' that lasts for several hours. After that you will experience a 'low' feeling or hangover effect that is a sign of withdrawal from the food: a feeling that will only be relieved by once more eating the food to which you have an intolerance.

A well-documented example of this reaction is the weekend headache or, in some cases, migraine that some people experience. They may have spent all week at work drinking perhaps five or six cups of coffee or tea each day. Then when the weekend comes and they have a few extra hours in bed they wake up with a headache that is only relieved when they have a drink of tea or coffee. These people have a caffeine addiction. They are kept on a constant high all week by the stimulus of coffee and have a 'hangover' at the weekend when they drink less of it or none at all.

The paradoxical nature of this type of food intolerance is that the very food you enjoy most or the food that is the staple of your diet could be the very food that is causing all the problems. That is one reason why these food intolerances are so hard to recognise and treat.

And one reason, of course, why people might not want to recognise them. They would rather put up with their headache or fatigue than give up their favourite chocolate or tea or biscuits and cake. Mere headache and fatigue are symptoms that accompany the early stages of food allergy. If the sufferer continues to put up with them and the underlying allergy is left undiagnosed the situation will get worse. The sufferer will develop a full-blown intolerance to foods and further symptoms will develop. In addition to headache and fatigue a bewildering variety of symptoms will appear – ringing in the ears, excessive sweating, irritable bowel syndrome, cold hands and feet, mental confusion and most common of all, a crabby feeling in the mornings.

It is this early morning fatigue that is a key indicator of food allergies. One patient with ME graphically described it: 'I feel so bad when I wake up I just don't even have the strength to roll over and look at my watch.'

When you think about it the reason for this is obvious. We have already described how food allergy can be like an addiction. If the sufferer does not keep the addiction topped up, he or she will experience withdrawal symptoms. So the person who is allergic to wheat, for instance, will find it very hard to get going in the mornings without that first slice of toast for breakfast.

Dr Theron Randolph, the well-known American expert on allergies, calls alcohol a 'jet-propelled food allergen'. Many alcoholic drinks, particularly whisky and beer, are made from grains and grains are the most common food allergen. Ingested in the form of alcohol they get into the system much faster, and somebody who is allergic to wheat, malt and barley will never get rid of this allergy if they continue to drink beer and whisky. This may be the major reason why ME sufferers find that even a small amount of alcohol makes their symptoms worse.

So if you think you have ME and the fatigue, brain fag and muddled thinking you are complaining about is worse in the morning and occurs for the most part only in the morning, then you must try and discover which foods might be causing your symptoms.

Do-it-yourself testing for food allergies is time consuming and demands great patience. If you have a pretty good idea which food or foods are causing your allergy it is fairly easy to test them. You stop eating the foods for at least five days. Then you try the food again. The reaction will be immediate this time because, after five days without the particular food, your body will have ceased to adapt to it and will react at once. If you have an acute reaction like stomach pains or severe headache it is likely that the food you have been avoiding is the allergen. You should then stop eating that food completely and try eating it again in a few months' time. Sometimes food allergies 'wear off' and you can eat the offending food in small amounts later on – sometimes after six months or a year.

The problem about self-testing is that it is hard to guess the foods which are causing the trouble. People often find it very difficult to understand that the foods they like most, and eat most often, are very likely to be the culprits. Clinical ecologists, those doctors that specialise in food allergy testing, confirm this time and time again in their patients. So if you are in the habit of eating the same thing, whether it is a bar of chocolate, a cheese sandwich or a cup of tea, to pick yourself up when you feel a bit low you must suspect that the food that is giving you that lift may be the very same food that is causing your problems. Many ME sufferers who have contacted the ME Action Campaign and the ME Association admit they cannot give up their regular cup of tea. Six or more times a day they perk themselves up with a cuppa. And each time, one or two hours later, they begin to feel awful and need another one.

We suggest that you start cutting out tea, coffee and other caffeinated drinks like fizzy colas. Many ME sufferers give up alcohol when they get this disease and if you have not done so you should give it a try.

Wheat and dairy products are among the commonest food allergens in this country and if you suspect these are at the root of your problem you should try cutting them out of your diet completely. The commonest visitor to the clinical ecologist is the fatigue sufferer whose favourite food is a cheese sandwich and a glass of milk, or a bowl of breakfast cereal.

You should stop eating wheat and other grains, dairy products including yoghurt, cheese, butter and cream for at least six days. You should also avoid any foods that contain these products, for instance, packet soups, pancakes, puddings, pies and pasta. If, especially on the third and fourth days, you feel really rough that is a good sign. This is a withdrawal symptom and it is evidence that your symptoms were indeed caused by foods that you were eating daily and have now cut out. At this stage you must resist all temptations to make yourself feel better by cheating on the diet. If you succumb to temptation you will ruin the whole test and will be back to square one.

By the fifth or sixth day you should be feeling quite a lot better. In fact you may feel better than you have done for months or even years. If you are, congratulations, you have made the first step to diagnosing your condition and doing something about it.

If you have no idea which foods might be causing your symptoms you have to take more drastic action – the exclusion diet or, perhaps, the Stone Age diet. It is wise to conduct an exclusion diet under the care of a qualified allergy specialist as reintroducing foods that are allergens can have nasty side effects and could be dangerous. It is also very difficult to stick to this regime if you are doing it on your own and you will need the support of a specialist.

The exclusion diet starts, ideally, with a five-day fast but this is probably only appropriate for people who are being tested in hospital or are confined to bed. If you feel you cannot fast then the Mansfield diet, named after leading allergist, Dr John Mansfield, might be more appropriate. This consists of lamb and pears, which have been found to be two of the least allergenic foods. You eat this for three meals a day for five days. During this time you eat no other food but make sure you avoid dehydration by drinking plenty of bottled spring water, at least eight glasses a day (tap water contains impurities that might hamper the test).

After five days of this diet you should be feeling fine, better than you have done for months, even if you had to go through a 'withdrawal' process in the first four days. If you do not feel any better it is unlikely that you have a food allergy. Five days is plenty of time for your body to get rid of any residues of allergenic foods so if you have symptoms after this time they will not be due to foods (although they could be due to chemicals or other things in your home or work environment such as gas, moulds or house dust).

The idea behind the Stone Age diet is that meat, fruit and vegetables are the foods least likely to cause food allergies. Man is thought to have eaten meat, fruit and vegetables for thousands of years and it is believed that these are our 'natural' foods. Cereals and sugars were only introduced into our diet in relatively recent history so it may be that we have not adapted to them as part of our natural diet.

If you are feeling better, you can start 'challenging' your body with different foods. The aim of this is to discover the foods that you can eat without harm and to build up a mixed, healthy diet. You should introduce foods back to the diet one at a time. And you should try only one new food a day. If you try more than that, symptoms from the first food may be obscured. On the first day after the fast or Stone Age diet you might try wholemeal bread for instance. Instead of eating meat for breakfast you would eat a piece of wholemeal bread and then if there is no reaction you should have some more bread for lunch and dinner. If you are testing a drink you should have it separately from the meal. If the food is a problem for you, you will normally experience symptoms within a few hours of eating it.

You should keep a detailed diary of what symptoms occur after eating each food and how long it is before they appear. Everyone varies in their allergic reactions to food. But a fairly common pathway of reaction is as follows:

Heartburn, indigestion and wind within half-an-hour of eating the food.

Headache, anxiety, feeling 'low' within an hour.

Bloated stomach or diarrhoea within three hours.

Hives and rashes within six to 12 hours.

Water retention causing a bloated feeling and weight gain in 12 to 15 hours.

Mouth ulcers, aching joints, aching muscles within two to four days.

You may not experience all of these symptoms but even if only one occurs after you have eaten a food it indicates an allergy.

Warning

If you experience a severe food reaction you should try drinking a tablespoon of sodium bicarbonate in a half-pint of warm water. This will produce diarrhoea and help you get rid of the offending food more quickly. (NB If you suffer from a heart condition you should not use this remedy as it can be dangerous – seek your doctor's advice instead.) Be warned that very rarely a food allergen can produce an extremely dangerous reaction – anaphylactic shock. If this happens you will have great difficulty breathing, you may become unconscious and you are in danger of dying. You will need immediate hospital treatment and the doctor who treats you should be told immediately what has caused this reaction. If you are testing foods it would be wise to have someone in the house who can help if such a reaction should occur. It is another very good reason why you should undergo food allergy testing under the care of a food allergy specialist.

If you find a food that causes symptoms you should stop eating it straight away and avoid it for several months. Later on, you can challenge yourself again with this food to see if it still causes a reaction. If it does not, you may start eating it again in very small amounts. By the end of testing, which can take several weeks of very hard work and perseverance, you should have a list of foods that you can eat without fear of allergic reaction.

If you have been testing for food allergy you must make sure the diet you will be eating is well balanced and nutritious. If you find you are limited to just a handful of foods, you risk not getting enough of the protein, carbohydrates, vitamins and minerals that you need and you should take supplements and seek expert advice from a clinical ecologist or nutritionist.

When testing foods you should try out other foods that might be a useful replacement. For instance, if you find you are allergic to cow's milk, try testing yourself against goat's milk, which may not have the same effect. If you find you are allergic to wheat, try testing yourself against alternatives like millet or oats. There are many alternative foods and if you do not try them you could find your lifestyle and eating habits severely restricted – and that takes all the pleasure out of food.

As we have said, testing yourself for food allergies can be very difficult; you may prefer to ask a doctor to help you. Getting this sort of help on the NHS is difficult as there are few NHS doctors who really understand allergies and are able to provide this service. You may like to visit a clinical ecologist, doctors who specialise in treating patients with food and chemical allergies. A list of clinical ecologists practising in this country can be obtained from Action Against Allergy or the British Society for Allergy and Environmental Medicine (see Appendix B for addresses).

Many of the food allergies we have discussed in this chapter occur because the food is eaten every single day at more than one meal. Today some allergists advise their patients to follow a rotation diet whereby you eat a wide variety of foods and not too much of any one kind of food, and leave a four-day gap between eating one food and then eating it again. So if you had oranges on a Monday you would then not eat oranges or citrus fruit again until the Friday. If you ate bread on a Tuesday you would not eat bread or wheat products again until Saturday.

The theory is that the four-day gap gives the body time to 'recover' from eating a particular food. Even if you have no allergy to a particular food we have seen that by eating the same food day-in, day-out you can develop allergies to the most innocuous foods: hence the rotation diet.

This diet can be very hard to stick to as it involves avoiding particular foods, and any foods that are in the same family or which might contain the same food. For instance if you ate wheat on a Monday you would have to avoid wheat and wheat products like cakes, breaded chicken drumsticks, meatballs, packet soups and any other foods that contain wheat flour, until Friday. That is not easy and means you have to read carefully the labels of every food you buy.

If you decide to follow the rotation diet you should start off by avoiding all the foods to which you showed an allergic reaction when tested. After two or three months you can try some of these foods again as very often the allergy 'wears off'. If this happens you can eat the food now and then, but do not go overboard and start eating the food every day or an allergic response is likely to develop all over again.

Other Allergy Tests

Fasting and then challenging yourself with different foods is not the only way to find out if you have an allergy. There are various tests available to pinpoint allergies and you should find out if these are available in your area.

The prick and scratch test: This was one of the first allergy tests to be developed but it is not widely used today because it is rather inaccurate. A small drop of the suspected allergen diluted in water is put onto the skin which is then scratched or pricked with a needle. The weal, red patch, that develops indicates whether the substance is an allergen.

Patch testing: This is fairly similar. The suspected allergens are placed on the skin and then taped down for several hours. If the skin reddens it indicates an allergy.

The RAST test: (Radio-allego-sorbent test) tests the blood to see if there are antibodies against foods, house dust mite and other possible allergens.

The cytotoxic test: Also a blood test but different to the RAST test. The white cells are removed from the patient's blood and then tested against foods and common chemicals. If there is an allergy the white cells are damaged and die and the severity of the allergy can be graded according to how quickly the white cells are destroyed.

The serial end-point skin titration test: Also called the Miller Method or provocation and neutralisation, this is a more sophisticated prick or scratch test. The allergen is injected into the skin to make a weal. If this grows over ten to fifteen minutes there is probably an allergy. If there is a reaction the patient is given a series of injections at ten-minute intervals of weaker and weaker concentrations of the allergen until the weal stops growing and the symptom, if there is one, stops completely. The doctors notes the dilution of allergen at which the reaction stopped. This is called the neutralising dose and is used in the treatment of the allergy. If the patient has a food allergy, a drop of the neutralising dose is placed under the tongue before meals and they can eat the food to which they are allergic with fewer, or no, symptoms. Sometimes the neutralising dose is given as an injection once or twice a week.

Sometimes this test is performed sublingually with drops placed under the tongue instead of given by injection.

Chemicals Allergies and How To Get Rid Of Them
Just as you may not realise you have a food allergy, you might not suspect you have what is called a chemical or environmental allergy. This is caused by a reaction to something in the environment – it might be petrol, or hairspray, or certain food additives, or toilet cleaner, photocopier chemicals, newsprint, paint, air freshener or pesticides.

As with food allergies, the initial exposure to a chemical might produce a reaction but the patient does not recognise the connection at the time. Gradually, the body adapts to the chemical by producing persistent symptoms and, rather like the 'addiction' to foods, the body becomes addicted to chemicals, often without realising it.

A good example of this kind of chemical addiction was seen in the case of a paint sprayer who suffered chronic migraine and depression for many years. One year he went on holiday to Eastbourne but within a few days was in severe pain with blinding headaches, fatigue and a general feeling of being ill. He tried to snap out of it by going for some fresh air along the sea front. When he walked along the pier he found his symptoms were considerably relieved, particularly at the point where the pier was being repainted. For the rest of the holiday he made sure he walked along the pier to get the fresh smell of paint that would make him feel better. He was addicted to chemicals released by fresh paint and when he was away from his job he suffered withdrawal symptoms that he could only relieve by smelling fresh paint.

Unfortunately, there are very few of us today who are lucky enough to have no contact at all with chemicals like paint, cigarette smoke and petrochemicals. It is also very difficult to assess which chemicals might be causing an allergic reaction when we use so many in our daily life.

There are two ways to tackle the problem. One is to visit a clinical ecologist who can test for chemicals and other substances such as pollen and house dust by injecting a minute amount into the arm and noting the reaction both in terms of weal growth and symptoms. Just as in the case of foods, neutralising drops can be provided which the patient takes under the tongue three times a day – an effective and painless way of reducing the symptoms produced by exposure to chemicals. The other way is to minimise your contact with chemicals in your everyday life.

If you smoke, or you live or work with a smoker, the chemicals from cigarettes may be to blame for some of your symptoms. Cigarettes give off hundreds of different chemicals any one of which can cause an allergic reaction. Many perfectly healthy people suffer headaches, stuffy nose, sore throat and watery eyes when sitting in a room with a smoker so it should come as no surprise that ME sufferers are particularly prey to the ill effects of cigarettes.

Ordinary household chemicals may also be the source of unpleasant chemical allergies. If you count up the number of chemicals you use to clean the house you might be shocked at the high number. You might have detergents, washing-up liquids, oven cleaner, toilet cleaner, bleach, disinfectant, furniture polish, window cleaner, floor polish, kettle descaler, dish-washing detergent, air freshener. That is a lot of household chemicals. It should be possible to halve this number at least. Ask yourself whether you really need all these things. Do you really need an air freshener when opening the windows and getting some fresh air would be just as effective and more pleasant? Do you really need a bleach and a disinfectant when they do much the same job?

When you have thrown away all your unnecessary chemicals you should transfer the ones you have left into glass bottles with tight-fitting lids (remember to label them carefully to avoid accidents). This will cut down the smells from these chemicals and as most household chemicals are stored in plastic containers it will cut down on the amount of 'plastic' chemicals kept in the house.

The same goes for toiletries that you might just take for granted. Do you use numerous shampoos, deodorants, hair-sprays, soaps, shaving foams without a second thought? You may be sensitive to any one of those. So to avoid a reaction throw out anything that is unnecessary and try to use natural ones such as those available from the Body Shop.

If you keep cans of paint and other DIY chemicals in the house, perhaps now is the time to invest in a garden shed to store them well away from your living area.

Gas and fuels that we use in heating and cooking may be a source of chemicals that produce allergic reactions in susceptible people. But it is rather expensive to test whether you are allergic to your cooker or your central heating so look at other things first.

Many people with chemical sensitivity have a very acute nose – they can smell things that other people cannot. You can put this nose to good use when thinking about what household chemicals might be causing your symptoms. If you go out into the fresh air and then come back into the house with a 'fresh' nose you should be able to sniff out the offending chemicals. Clinical ecologists know that anything you can smell very acutely or do not like the smell of is probably a problem for you. However, if you have been living with the same chemicals for many years you may not notice their smells anymore.

It will take an independent observer to notice, and it is for this reason that Dr Jean Monro, who runs her own allergy and environmental medicine hospital, employs a specialist in environmental medicine, Philip Barlow, to go into the homes of patients with chemical allergies and inspect them for possible chemical contamination.

Many people are sensitive to petrol and car fumes and this can be very unpleasant if you live in a city or have to drive every day. Filling up the tank with petrol can be particularly aggravating for susceptible people and having a garage attached to the house can also be the source of nasty fumes lingering in the home.

The chemicals that are added to food, whether by accident or by design in the case of food additives or pesticides, may also cause considerable distress. Sometimes these can be quite baffling. For instance, one sufferer, who could eat apples one week and then developed a marked reaction the next, found that she had a sensitivity to a particular pesticide that was used by some farmers.

It is virtually impossible to avoid contact with all twentieth century chemicals but it is certainly possible to minimise it by just taking basic precautions. You might even find you can cope as long as you have a 'safe haven' like a bedroom in your house that is an oasis away from chemicals.

Some of the actions suggested in this chapter may sound a little extreme but most of them are really quite sensible. After all, do we really want to go on eating a food that makes us ill or breathing in chemicals that make us go into a decline?

For ME sufferers whose health is very bad the allergy connection is particularly important. Some patients can hardly get up except to go to the bathroom. They are confined to their bedroom almost 24 hours a day. For them it is particularly important to look at their bedroom and their whole house from an environmental point of view. If they feel better in another room they should switch rooms. If they always feel better when visiting friends or when they are outside in the fresh air they should suspect there may be something about their house that is contributing to their symptoms. This could be, for instance, an undetected gas leak, or formaldehyde from cavity wall insulation. We are not saying that allergies cause ME, but we are saying that patients with ME often develop allergies and that sometimes their health problems can be traced to a single chemical exposure which significantly changes their immune system.

8 The Candida Connection

An approach to ME that has received considerable publicity is the combination of diet and drugs to eliminate *Candida albicans*. Although Candida does not cause ME, many patients, particularly women, almost certainly suffer from an overgrowth of this organism. And many patients who think they have ME may actually be suffering from the symptoms of Candida as the two conditions can be very similar.

Many NHS doctors do not recognise it as a real problem because it is only in the last few years, largely through the efforts of American doctors, William Crook and Orian Truss, that the importance of Candida as a disease organism has begun to be recognised. So the information will not yet have made its way to the medical textbooks. If you are lucky you will have an enlightened doctor who will have heard of Candida and its effects on the human body and who will be prepared to help you get rid of it. If not, there are some ways you can fight this infection yourself.

Candida albicans is a type of yeasty fungus that inhabits everybody's bowel – we probably become infected during birth simply by passing down our mother's birth canal. Spores of various fungi are all around us, in the air and on our food, so simple contact with the world means we ingest fungi all the time. Candida is not normally a problem because it is kept under control by the beneficial bacteria that also live in the gut, and by a healthy immune system.

But if the immune system is impaired, or the numbers of beneficial bacteria are depleted, Candida can grow out of control producing a range of symptoms. In patients suffering severe immunosuppression such as AIDS, or after aggressive drug treatment for cancer, Candida can actually be the cause of death. If it gets really out of control in these patients it can infect other organs of the body, even the brain, where it becomes extremely difficult to treat. But in ME sufferers things rarely progress to that stage.

Candida is normally quite harmless but when it is allowed to grow out of control it will try and colonise any area of the body that is warm and moist, such as the gut and the vagina, and can cause a wide range of symptoms.

Women who have taken the contraceptive pill for any length of time and anyone who has taken repeated courses of antibiotics or steroids such as cortisone or prednisolone will be vulnerable to Candida overgrowth. Antibiotics tend to change the normal bacterial consituents of the gut allowing the yeast to proliferate. They actually kill all the good bacteria as well as the harmful bacteria that they are prescribed for, leaving this yeast to run riot. Many ME sufferers are people who have had repeated courses of broad spectrum antibiotics such as tetracycline and they are at risk because their immune system does not work properly and they seem to be unable to control the Candida growth.

It has been estimated that as many as 50 per cent of ME patients might have problems with Candida and this will exacerbate the symptoms of ME and make it more difficult to recover. With Candida you are battling against two diseases, not just one.

Candida can cause a wide range of symptoms, both from direct contact with the gut and vagina, and by releasing toxins into the blood stream that interfere with a range of bodily functions. Some signs of Candida are oral and vaginal thrush, heartburn, wind, indigestion, mucus in the stools, constipation, colic, a bloated abdomen, headache, muscle and joint pains, fatigue and depression, loss of memory and concentration, weight fluctuations, loss of libido and cystitis.

These are a very wide range of symptoms and many of them are indentical with those of ME. It is this similarity of symptoms that makes us think many ME patients are not, in fact, suffering from ME but think they are because the symptoms are the same and they may not have heard of Candida in the glare of publicity about ME. If they did but know it, Candida is often the major problem. If their Candida was eliminated, along with the food allergies that often go with it, they would get much better.

Diagnosis of Candida, or candidiasis as it is sometimes called, is difficult because there are no tests that will identify an overgrowth. Since we are all infected with Candida it is difficult to pinpoint those people who have more than everyone else. If your practitioner recognises Candida as a problem the diagnosis will be made on your clinical symptoms and whether you respond to Candida treatment.

It is worth noting that clinical ecologists, nutritionists and naturopaths are more likely to be able to recognise Candida problems than the normal GP. In this country the study of nutrition (and this would include information on Candida) gets very low priority during medical training and most medical schools do not have separate nutrition courses. So it is not surprising that family doctors do not know about these subjects.

If you have a mild Candida problem you are likely to respond to an anti-Candida diet. If the infection is more severe you will be prescribed anti-fungal drugs that clear the infection, and you will be put on an anti-Candida diet to make sure it does not come back.

The two most commonly prescribed anti-Candida drugs are nystatin (brand name Nystan) and oral amphotericine B (brand name Fungilin). If you are given either of these drugs you will be put on a six-week trial to see if they are having any effect and if it is worth carrying on. Treatment might last six months or up to a year to make sure all the Candida is killed.

Most doctors will start you off on a low dose of nystatin and build up to a higher dose. This is to avoid a severe reaction to toxins produced by yeasts as they die off. At the beginning of the treatment your body will be exposed to poisons given off by the Candida as it dies off. This is called the Herxheimer reaction. These poisons might make you feel even worse for a while but gradually this should pass and you will eventually feel a lot better. The dose might be increased from half-a-tablet a day to start with gradually up to eight tablets a day and then taper off to a maintenance dose of one or two tablets a day. Nystatin is also available in a powder form that is thought to be more efficient as it is dispersed more evenly through the alimentary tract. Some people may experience side effects such as nausea, vomiting and diarrhoea when the drug is used at high doses.

There is a lot of controversy surrounding anti-fungal therapy. There are no clear guideline on how long it takes to kill all the yeast. Although these drugs are said to be very safe, as they are not absorbed through the gut into the body, it is unlikely that anyone would want to be on permanent drug therapy of any kind. Taking an anti-fungal drug for too long may also give rise to problems with resistance. The Candida may 'get used' to the drug and you will need a higher dose to keep it under control or the Candida may evolve to become resistant to the drug altogether. For these reasons it would probably be unwise to take the treatment for more than two years.

The best way to avoid Candida overgrowth is to prevent it and you can do this by going on an anti-Candida diet. If you are taking drugs to kill the Candida you should go on this diet at the same time. You are defeating the purpose of the drugs if you carry on feeding the yeast.

Yeasts, as any breadmaker or home brewer will know, feed on sugar. So your first defence against Candida is to stop eating sugar, particularly refined sugars that the Candida can pounce on as soon as you swallow them. Syrup, honey, white sugar on your cereal, jam, the sugar in cakes and biscuits, chocolates, sweets, sweet drinks, the sugar added to convenience foods – all will have to go. This sounds drastic and it is. Until now you probably did not realise just how many of your everyday foods contained sugar and they are all feeding your Candida. So start reading the labels of every food you buy and watch out for that hidden sugar.

Some Candida experts also recommend giving up foods that contain yeast or yeasty products as Candida is thought to feed on other yeasts and fungi. There are many yeasty foods including bread and bread products, mushrooms, Marmite, cheeses, soured cream, wine and beer, vinegars and pickles made with vinegar. You will have to stop eating these as well.

This is a very strict diet and you might find it too much all in one go. The best way to adapt is to start off by cutting out all sugars. Once you have done that successfully you can start to concentrate on the yeasty foods by finding a yeast-free whole-grain bread substitute, for instance soda bread, rice cakes or oatcakes.

There are a number of dietary supplements that are said to help the treatment of Candida which you can take while on the anti-Candida diet. Probiotics are concentrated cultures of bacteria such as *Lactobacillus acidophilus* that normally live in the gut and help to fight hostile organisms like Candida. 'Live' yoghurt also contains these beneficial bacteria and by eating this and taking supplements such as Probion you will boost the numbers of these beneficial bacteria – which will help fight the Candida. You may need to take supplements of vitamin K if you are prone to Candida overgrowth. The bacteria in the small bowel produce some of the vitamin K that is absorbed through the gut wall for our own use, and if the numbers of bacteria are depleted this source of vitamin K is also reduced. If you have a depressed immune system you may need extra supplements of minerals, like zinc, and other vitamins to boost your capacity to fight these infections. These are discussed more fully in Chapter 15.

Garlic is an effective anti-fungal agent and is said to help build up the immune system to fight disease as well.

If you are a woman who has problems with vaginal thrush, you can ask you doctor for pessaries of an anti-fungal drug that you use for a few days to clear the infection. After that you should try and prevent further infection by making sure you dry yourself properly after a shower or bath. Everytime you go to the toilet make sure you wipe yourself from front to back to avoiding transferring Candida from the gut to the vagina. It is probably better to have showers than baths as this stops you soaking in nice warm water that Candida loves. If you do have a bath, throw in a handful of salt instead of using a bubble bath which can be an irritant that will exacerbate the effects of the infection. The salt changes the acid balance of the water and helps prevent the Candida proliferating.

If you have cystitis read Dr Patrick Kingsley's *Conquering Cystitis* which will tell you more about the cystitis–Candida connection.

The Candida theries are fairly new and many doctors may not be sympathetic if you demand a prescription for nystatin. Stay calm and explain why you think Candida may be at the root of some of your problems. If your doctor is still not convinced show him or her any information or books (see Appendix A) you may have on Candida; your doctor may not have realised how important it can be.

Many ME sufferers feel remarkably better after a course of anti-Candida therapy and it is well worth a try if many of your ME symptoms, particularly the cerebral ones and those affecting the gut, are identical to those for Candida. You are more likely to suffer Candida if you are a woman but men can suffer from Candida overgrowth too. If your major symptoms are fatigue and muscle pains but you have none of the bloating, indigestion, wind or mental confusion then it is unlikely that Candida is a problem for you.

9 The Psychological Symptoms: anti-depressants, self-help groups and keeping a diary

The physical symptoms of ME are inextricably bound up with a wide range of psychological problems that make the illness very hard to deal with, both for doctors and patients. Every sufferer will remember the times of self-pity, depression and loneliness that seem inevitably to go hand-in-hand with ME. Not all of these things are caused by the organic disease. Some of the psychological problems may be caused by the problem of having a doctor who refuses to recognise the illness, or a disbelieving spouse, or friends who give up their friendship because you are always ill. It can be the most dispiriting thing in the world to have a disease that few people believe in and you cannot seem to recover from.

Learning to recognise the psychological problems associated with ME will equip you to handle them more effectively, but the first step is to recognise that these feelings are normal. Every ME sufferer will tell you he or she has been depressed, lonely, paranoid or just plain fed-up with the whole world. So you are not the only one who has ever experienced these feelings and they are nothing to be ashamed of.

Unfortunately, the psychological aspects of ME have helped to reinforce the view that it is a disease of the mind. But there are many other physical illnesses that are marked by depression. People with brain tumours, heart disease and senile dementia all suffer depression as normal symptoms of their disease yet they are not dismissed by their doctors as hysterics or hypochondriacs.

Some doctors debate as to whether the viral infection comes first, followed by emotional ills as part of the illness, or whether the patient's emotional state predisposes them to succumb to a viral infection. This is not so easy to resolve as there is good evidence for both sides of the argument. It is well known that people under a lot of emotional stress, for instance, going through a divorce or bereavement or just a hard time at work, are not able to combat infections as well as people with fewer stresses.

The immune system seems to become damaged by stress so that it is not so well able to fight disease. A good example of this has been seen in breast cancer where a significant proportion of the women who develop breast cancer have experienced a traumatic life event, such as a divorce or bereavement, in the previous five years compared with women who do not develop breast cancer. In America there is evidence that people under a lot of stress are more likely to succumb to the virus that causes infectious mononucleosis. Their emotional state seems to predispose them to viral infection and prolonged recovery.

Alternatively, it could be the illness itself that produces the emotional abnormalities seen in ME sufferers as it does in brain tumours or heart disease. Even if the initial viral infection does not produce such effects the social consequences of ME will almost certainly influence the psyche. However, these arguments are academic. What matters is that most ME patients suffer from emotional disturbances and need to recognise what they are in order to overcome them.

Psychological or, more accurately 'cerebral' symptoms are part and parcel of the disease process of ME. The infecting virus not only affects the muscles, causing myalgia and fatigue, but it is thought to get into the central nervous system, the brain and the spinal cord. It may even get into the tiny nerves that line the inside of the skin, which may account for the strange pins and needles sensations that many sufferers report. If the nervous system is particularly affected, then it is quite likely that psychological symptoms will dominate over the physical ones. Whereas if the virus has more severely affected the muscles, it will be the physical symptoms that cause more trouble.

While many of the psychological symptoms are an organic part of the disease process itself, the situation may be further complicated by a set of reactive psychological symptoms – those that occur as a reaction to having ME. You may feel anxious about having ME, or depressed at not being able to predict the outcome of the disease, or unhappy that you cannot do the things in life that you had planned. As the symptoms and treatment of both the psychological and reactive aspects of ME are the same, there is no point in trying to separate which symptoms are caused by what. The important thing is to treat them and learn to cope with them.

Depression

Depression is one of the symptoms of ME and it may also be the hardest to deal with because it can be difficult for sufferers to recognise just how depressed they are. It is not unique to ME sufferers; every single person in the world suffers depression at some point in their life – it is a normal, healthy reaction to some of life's problems.

It is not unusual to become down occasionally about having ME and it would be very surprising if an ME sufferer did not experience depression. What is dangerous is when that depression occurs all the time or there is no obvious reason for it. The feelings of despair that sweep over you can be suffocating. When you experience depression you will only be able to see the negative aspects of life lost in a long black tunnel of despair at the end of which there seems to be no light. Life might not feel worth living, you may feel a burden to your family, you will feel tired of being sick and sick of being tired. You might feel stretched to the limits of physical and emotional endurance by ME.

This type of despair is dangerous. If you get to this state you must seek help. Depression has a knack of distorting all your feelings and your thinking so that you can no longer make rational decisions. Your mind will no longer think logically so that actions you would have abhorred when you were well seem perfectly acceptable to you when you are ill.

There are no statistics on the number of suicides that are a direct result of ME. Dr Melvin Ramsay knows of six ME patients who have felt so totally depressed by their disease that they have felt suicide was the only way out. In 1969 he diagnosed ME in a 12-year-old boy whose mother also had ME: 'Ten years later, at the age of 22 and a student at Reading University, he was still struggling with the aftermath of the disease, which took the form of complete reversal of sleep rhythm, when sheer despair drove him to suicide by taking an overdose of nitrazepam.'

Dr Jean Monro had a patient from the West country who had suffered from ME for six or seven years and at the age of 32 killed himself with a shotgun. A friend of the family of one of the patients whose case history is recounted at the end of the book committed suicide with an overdose of sleeping pills – he had had ME for four years.

It would be impossible to predict whether these and other suicides could have been prevented if there had been adequate help available. But that help is available if you look for the warning signs and seek help before the problems become insurmountable on your own.

Utter despair is not the only symptom of depression. Other signs to be alert for are weepiness, loss of interest in family, friends and things you used to enjoy, loss of appetite, low self-esteem, feelings of guilt, pessimism, irritability, and disturbed sleep, particularly waking up early.

In general practice most doctors would include fatigue as one of the ways of diagnosing depression. But in ME fatigue is so much a part of the physical illness that it cannot be used as a useful guideline.

Anxiety

Anxiety is that panicky feeling of being on edge. It is similar to the feeling you might experience just before going on stage to act or before standing up to speak in public. However, in those situations the anxiety normally passes fairly quickly and can even give you that extra edge to cope with the situation.

Anxiety is not helpful when it lasts a long time. The main symptoms are feelings of nervousness and agitation. You may find the palms of your hands sweat, your mouth becomes dry, your heart pounds and your bowel become irritable. This is not a very comfortable condition to live with as it is virtually impossible to relax in this state. Anxiety often occurs with depression and it can be difficult to distinguish between the two conditions.

Paranoia

Sometimes feelings of suspicion and wariness of those around you might develop. This is another psychological problem that occurs as a reaction to ME. Anyone with a long-term illness like ME naturally wants to be able to talk about it to relatives and friends. ME can become an all-consuming way of life to the sufferer but what she or he has to remember is that there is a life outside ME. While you might want to talk about your illness to relatives and friends they may have become bored of hearing about it and may start to distance themselves from you.

This can be unkind and rather upsetting and you may feel that they are doing it because they do not like you anymore. That is probably not the case; they may just not want to hear about ME whenever they see you. Either you have to find people who do want to talk about ME or should find something else to talk about with these people. If you dwell on it too much, you may become very isolated and start to believe that they hate you for your illness. If you have these feelings of paranoia you must recognise that they are quite natural and probably arise because you feel you have no one you can talk to. This is where ME support groups are so important and they are discussed at the end of the chapter.

Organic Brain Symptoms
Most of these symptoms can be attributed to the fact that your nervous system is in some way affected by the viral infection.

Many ME sufferers have a whole range of symptoms that can be described as emotional lability. People who were normally of an even temperament before they contracted ME might now fly into a rage at the slightest incident: something that will give them the unfair reputation of being 'touchy'.

Others who were once very resilient in their ability to take criticism might now find themselves extremely hurt by the slightest reprimand. People who would have described themselves as unemotional might find they now cry easily at sentimental films. Antonia, formerly a television producer, says: 'Nowadays, the slightest criticism really stings me to the quick even though, if I were to be objective about it, I would probably acknowledge the criticism was never intended as such. Conversely, even the slightest praise almost brings tears to my eyes and I feel absurdly full of warmth for the person who praised me.'

One of the most distressing things about this emotional lability is that it is very difficult to control. This is not only upsetting for the sufferer but for the relatives and friends who might not know what to expect next.

You may also be more clumsy than before, you may reach out for things and miss them or drop them. You may call things by the wrong name, for instance the cat might become the dog or the baby might become the pram, or you may mispronounce words or spell them incorrectly. Co-ordination becomes affected, for instance driving a car can be slightly affected, making it more difficult to reverse into a parking space or do a three-point turn.

Loss of memory and concentration are two symptoms that can be directly attributed to the effects of the viral infection on the brain cells. Many ME sufferers discover that they are forgetful and have a very poor short-term memory; they cannot remember things that were mentioned only a short time ago. Shopping lists and phone numbers are often instantly forgotten and the sufferer finds him or herself writing everything down so that it cannot be overlooked. If you previously had a very good memory for names and faces you may find you can no longer fit the name to the face.

Loss of concentration is closely related to the loss of memory that so many sufferers report and it can be extremely frustrating not to be able to follow a conversation or a radio or television programme. Since ME is a very passive disease it can be hard to fill the 24 hours in a day when you cannot even concentrate on something for more than ten to 15 minutes. Even reading a book can become a major hurdle as you find yourself reading the same sentence over and over again to get the gist of what is going on only to find that once over the page you have forgotten the plot.

Although short-term memory is severely affected in some people the long-term memory does not seem to suffer. So you will still remember events from before ME. There are no recorded cases of ME sufferers who have become total amnesiacs.

How To Cope With Psychological Problems

The first step in coping with the psychological problems of ME is to recognise that they are there.

If you or your family feel your depression or anxiety has reached a crisis then go to your doctor for help. Do not be afraid to tell him or her about your feelings as this will give useful clues as to what drug should be prescribed. While most ME sufferers would be wise to avoid unnecessary drug treatment this is an exception. Anti-depressants can be very useful in getting you over a crisis in your illness and, as long as you and your doctor recognise that the treatment will be short term, there should be no problem in using these drugs.

The Rev. Michael Mayne, author of an account of ME called '*A Year Lost and Found*' said 'I haven't been depressed, I'm one of the lucky ones.' But he was given anti-depressants in September 1986 and was still on them nearly two years later. He attributes some of his recovery to them.

When you visit the doctor for depression he or she will consider three main classes of drugs for treatment: these are the tricyclic anti-depressants, novel (or atypical) anti-depressants or monoamine oxidase inhibitors (MAOIs). They all work by modifying the effects of certain natural chemicals in the brain (monamines). Since these chemicals also occur outside the brain these drugs may have side effects.

You may have heard of lithium as a treatment for depression. This is generally reserved for the treatment of manic depressives who have episodes of severe depression alternating with bouts of elation and frenetic activity but this is not the type of depression seen in ME.

The tricyclic anti-depressants include imipramine, amitrypty-line, desipramine, dothiepin, and nortryptiline, and they are the most commonly used. They have been in use for about 20 years and are generally very effective. But some of the side effects of the tricyclics can be just the same as the symptoms of ME, the commonest being dry mouth, blurred vision, constipation, occasionally difficulties in passing urine, dizziness and drowsiness. Some patients may find their hands shake slightly or they become sweaty. If you have any of these symptoms as part of your ME you should tell your doctor as this might affect the choice of drug in treating your depression.

The novel anti-depressants are chemically different from the tricyclics and include mianserin, maprotilene, and trazodone. When these drugs were first introduced they were hailed as an improvement because they had fewer effects outside the brain and so there were fewer side effects. However some doctors feel they do not work as well as the tricyclics and the side effects, when they do occur, seem to be more severe.

The MAOIs are often prescribed when the other types of anti-depressant do not work. They include phenelzine and tranylcypromine and can sometimes cause a drop in blood pressure making the patient feel dizzy, although this feeling normally passes after a while. The major drawback of the MAOIs is that a number of foods have to be avoided while taking them. Patients have to avoid, in particular, cheese, Marmite, and red wine or they will experience a dangerous drop in blood pressure. If your doctor prescribes MAOIs you will be given a card listing all the foods you must not eat. You must also avoid ALL other drugs or medicines, even those bought over the counter at the chemist, unless your doctor has cleared them first.

Most of these drugs are taken as tablets or capsules in a once daily dose and are usually prescribed for several months. Even if the depression lifts in the first few weeks of treatment, many doctors will advise you to carry on with the full course as there is considerable evidence to show you are less likely to suffer a relapse if treatment is continued for around six months. Sometimes the beneficial effects of the treatment will take a few weeks to appear but the side effects might start straightaway. Many of the side effects will subside after a few weeks and depending on which you are suffering from your doctor may or may not recommend you persevere with the treatment. You must always tell your doctor about any side effects as they may be important.

Drug treatment of anxiety is fraught with difficulties as most of the drugs that have been the cornerstone of treatment for many years are potentially addictive. The benzodiazepine tranquillizers, which include diazepam (Valium) and lorazepam (Ativan), will relieve anxiety in the first six weeks of use but after that there is usually no effect. Side effects include drowsiness and lethargy and loss of concentration. But the really big problem with these drugs is dependence bordering on true addiction.

It is estimated that one in every three people who take these tranquillizers continuously for more than six months will experience extremely unpleasant withdrawal symptoms including anxiety and insomnia (the very symptoms the drugs were prescribed for in the first place), panic attacks, poor memory or concentration. Some suffer loss of appetite while others feel ravenously hungry. Constipation, diarrhoea, headaches, muscle aches and pains, blurred vision, sensitivity to light and loud noises are all commonly reported. These side effects can sometimes persist for more than a year.

It is unlikely that your doctor will prescribe benzodiazepine tranquillizers nowadays. As you can see from the list of side effects, many of the symptoms are very similar to those of ME. If you were trying to withdraw from a benzodiazepine how would you know if these symptoms were side effects or your disease?

When your problem is anxiety some doctors will try you on an anti-depressant as some of these drugs have anti-anxiety properties and seem to be less habit forming than the benzodiazepines. Some of the anti-depressants also have sedative properties and for the patient who has disturbed sleep patterns anti-depressants can be invaluable in establishing a regular sleep pattern.

It is not the purpose of this book to recommend drug therapy in general – too many GPs prescribe drugs only too readily and usually without the in-depth consultation the ME patient needs.

But drugs can be very useful in a crisis and we will return to the subject of anti-depressants in Chapter 13.

Self Help
There are some things that every sufferer can do to help themselves out of the rut of depression, anxiety and the other psychological symptoms that are often a part of ME.

One of the first things you can do is to get in touch with other ME sufferers. The ME Association has a wide network of self-help groups throughout the country and they will put you in touch with other sufferers in your area (see the address in Appendix B).

Getting in touch with other ME sufferers will help you put your illness in perspective. If, until now, you have been struggling along on your own you might feel you are the only one in the world to experience such an awful disease. Joining a group will make you realise that other people have the same symptoms and many will have ones that sound even worse than yours. Probably the greatest benefit of joining a group is being able to talk about your problem without getting the feeling that the people who are listening to you are getting bored. People who are healthy are unlikely to want to sit and listen to details of your illness for any length of time but a fellow sufferer will be more willing.

Another plus of joining a group is that you are more likely to listen and learn from the experiences of other sufferers. Many people find it easier to follow a friend's advice, particularly if they also have ME, than the advice of a well-meaning doctor who has no personal experience of the disease.

Finding out as much about your illness as possible is also a good way of taking some control of it. The more you know about ME the more prepared you will be for any relapses or new symptoms that might occur along the path to recovery. Reading this book is a good start but with any 'new' disease there will be new research starting all the time so make sure you stay in touch with its progress.

Keeping a diary
Keeping a diary is a very good way of monitoring the progress of your recovery. While you might feel at your lowest ebb for many months it could be that you are not as bad as you have been in the past. Having a diary to look back on will help you realise that you are making progress even if it feels like a long and tortuous route.

Ideally, your diary should record all your symptoms and detail how often they occurred and how severe they were. For instance, you might write that even peeling the potatoes was too much for you or that you could walk 100 yards before feeling faint. It will also help to record what foods you have been eating. If you suspect you might have a food allergy this will give you some idea of which foods might be the culprits.

Some symptoms, like depression, are very difficult to describe in words so you might like to use a method employed by many doctors for getting patients to describe the severity of symptoms over a long period of time. If you draw a five inch long line on a blank piece of paper, the left-hand end might represent the worst you have ever been while the right-hand would be the best you have ever been. You then make a mark on the line to indicate how you feel today. If you are assessing tiredness, for instance, and today you feel almost as bad as your worst day, the mark would be close to the left-hand end. But if you are scoring for headache and you are feeling fairly well the mark would be towards the right-hand end. By measuring the distance from the left-hand end to your mark over a period of time you get a good graphic representation of how your symptoms are progressing. The technique sounds deceptively simple but it really does help.

Keeping a diary is fairly time consuming and some days you might not feel up to it. But if you do manage to it can be a real boost to you during difficult times. It can be reassuring to read that your condition has improved overall compared with one or two years ago even though you might feel slightly worse than you did two weeks ago.

10 Employment and ME

If you meet a stranger at a party virtually the first thing he will ask is 'What do you do?' We tend to define people by their jobs, so someone is a teacher, or a journalist, or a builder, or a secretary.

In our society if someone is unemployed they lack an identity. If someone is unemployed *and* has a mysterious viral infection they lack more than an identity. They are slightly strange as well.

There is great pressure put on everyone to work, to earn their living, to contribute to society. But if you have ME it is quite likely that you will have had to give up work and when you give it up not only do you give up earning money, you also lose a certain amount of status in society. If you become unemployed with ME suddenly all the roles change. You might feel you are no longer a valuable citizen but a handicapped burden who needs to be looked after by other people. You might feel guilty and feel you have no confidence or self-esteem left. With those feelings added to the burden of having ME, life can be tough. But there are ways of overcoming this.

Unfortunately society has a problem with illness. If you are ill you are weak, and very few people will readily admit to weakness. Everyone knows of those who refuse to succumb when they are ill and struggle into work with a raging temperature when they really should be at home in bed. Not only do they make themselves feel worse but they probably infect the whole office with their germs. If only society could accept that admitting you were ill and staying in bed for a few days does not make you a worse person but might make you better very much more quickly.

In the early stages of ME it is quite likely that you might have spent several months struggling to cope with getting to work and keeping up with the workload. After about six months of constant fatigue and feeling unwell all the time your work will have started to suffer. You might have difficulty in concentrating, difficulty in making decisions, and find it hard to remember things. You will probably be a regular visitor to the doctor and have had to take a lot of time off work. Your colleagues are probably starting to wonder what is happening to you and your boss certainly will be.

It is at this stage that you will have to stop and take stock of the situation. It's decision time. Are you going to stay at work or try working part-time? Can you cope with work and ME or should you concentrate full time on getting better? How will your finances stand up to you being unemployed? Should you struggle on until sickness benefit from your employer runs out or make a clean break? What sacrifices will you and your family have to make if you do give up work?

All these question and many more will have to be answered. It is going to be hard to deal with them and the stress of making these decisions could very well make your ME worse for a while. But they are things that have to be resolved. If you are struggling on, trying to hold down a full-time job and coping with ME at the same time something will eventually give. It is far better to sit down and work out these problems than to wait until there is a crisis. It will probably have become obvious by now that things cannot carry on as they are. You have got to make the choice. Is work more important or your health?

Deciding to give up your job because of ME is a tough decision to make. But you are not alone. Thousands of ME sufferers have had to give up work because of their disease. Many of the people caught up in the ME outbreaks described in earlier chapters had to give up work through ill health. Ten of the 59 nurses involved in the outbreak at the hospital in Durban, South Africa in 1955 had to retire from their jobs as three years afterwards they still had disabilities caused by their illness.

The decision to give up work does not come lightly and is particularly difficult for ME sufferers as they tend to be people who have worked hard in order to achieve an impressive work record. Losing a job, whether it is your own decision or your employer's, is a major life event. It will be a very stressful period for you as you try and come to terms with no longer having a job and, you may feel, no longer having an identity. But if your illness has meant you have really struggled to hold down your job, then becoming unemployed could be a blessing in disguise. It will give you a chance to try and recover properly from ME without the strains of keeping a job.

Research into the health of the unemployed has shown they suffer more ill health and higher death rates than the rest of the population. While some of this can be attributed to higher levels of smoking among unemployed people, the stress of being out of work, looking for a job and being short of money can all take their toll. These worries have to be added to those of having a disease like ME. As an ME sufferer you have two choices. You can wallow in your misery, become more depressed and lose interest in the world or you can drag yourself out of the pit.

When you first stop work the only thing you are likely to want to do is rest and sleep. Over the past few months you have probably struggled to keep your job and that is exhausting. You might feel any of a range of emotions: self-pity, shock, disbelief, guilt, anger. This is natural and is part of the grieving process that you go through. After all, you have just been forced to give up something that was an important part of your life and exchanging a well-established routine for the unknown can be scary.

After about four to six weeks of this torpor, and presuming that this length of rest has cleared your mind, you will be ready to start thinking of the future. It would be unwise to make any big decisions while you are still getting over the loss of your job. You are unlikely to make rational decisions while you are still in such a state of uncertainty. Wait until you are in a better frame of mind. This is the time to start reassessing your life and your illness; to start thinking about what you want from life and perhaps to change your priorities.

Not many people have the chance to take a step back and think about themselves and their lives, they probably never have the chance to sit down and think about life or even to get to know themselves. As an ME sufferer who is not working you have this chance. While it may not sound like much at the moment it could be the only opportunity you will ever have to find yourself.

If you do give up work you will have to revise all your ideas about what gives you fulfilment and enjoyment out of life. If you have been used to measuring your worth by what you achieve at work you will take time to adjust to the idea that there is more to life than work or money. You will have to find other things that give you a sense of self-esteem. While you have ME, activities that you barely thought about before you were ill such as gardening, knitting or jigsaws might give you more satisfaction than you had ever imagined.

You will only feel that sense of accomplishment if you set tasks that are within your capabilities. Do not dwell on what you used to be capable of doing but focus on what you can do now. Be realistic about your limitations and avoid setting lofty goals that will make you feel worse when you cannot achieve them.

It is important to focus on your inner worth. Who you are is much more important than what you are. By enduring ME and learning to cope with it you are developing your character to a depth that most other people will never attain. You might find you have hidden qualities of patience, understanding and self-control that you had never dreamed were there. At the time, enduring pain and suffering and losing things that are important to you make you want to curl up in a corner and escape from the world, but when it is all over you will look back on the experience and recognise that it was not all bad, that there were some things you could salvage, that you could say made you a 'better' person.

It is important not to let other people ruin your own self-esteem. It does not matter what anyone else thinks about you and your illness. They are not the ones having to cope with it – you are. Keep in mind that you are the strong and brave one because you are living with a disease for which there is no easy solution.

If you feel you cannot bear to give up work, then there are certain changes you are going to have to make to your lifestyle. If work is all-important you will have to give up other things in life and your family will probably have to take second place. If you want to make a success of your working life there are several things you can do to help.

One of these is to stop all unnecessary exertion. Don't stand when you can sit and don't sit when you can lie down sums this up admirably. If you want to concentrate on work you will have to do everything you can to save enough energy for it. That probably means sleeping all weekend to recover from the week's work and gather enough strength for Monday morning. It means getting home each evening, eating and going straight to bed. It means cancelling all social engagements. You cannot work hard and play hard with ME – it's either one or the other. Telephone people instead of going to see them in their office. If you have a job that involves a lot of physical work think about changing it, or ask your employers for a transfer to something less demanding on your physical energy. Try and organise your time so that you are more efficient. For instance, if you are going to get some stationery out of the cupboard, do another task like photo-copying at the same time so you only have to get up from your desk once.

All these things may seem a bit excessive. They are. But if you are determined to keep your job they are essential. If you want to keep on working you will have to recognise that you will probably have no energy left for doing anything else. Some ME sufferers do manage to keep their jobs and maybe even succeed in being promoted but generally it is at the expense of their home and social life. For many ME sufferers family and friends are more important.

If you cannot continue in your present job you might feel a change of employment would suit you. There are plenty of opportunities for retraining and moving into new areas. But before you make the commitment to a new job you have to be totally honest with yourself. Are you going to be able to cope with it? Remember that a new employer may not be so sympathetic to your condition as the employer you spent some time with and worked hard for. Do you really want a new job or are you just putting off the decision to give up work altogether because you cannot bear to contemplate the consequences of unemployment?

If you are determined to do some sort of work or your condition has considerably improved you may feel ready to do some part-time work. Your old employer might be sympathetic to the idea and you may even be able to find someone to share the job with. Do not take just any part-time job simply because it is an offer of work. Many part-time jobs, for instance shop work, are too physically demanding. It is important to find a job that you know you will be able to do because it will be very disappointing for you if you then find you cannot. Of course you do not have to get a job that pays. You might think of doing part-time voluntary work where there are fewer rules about what time you have to turn up and how many hours a week you have to work.

Sickness And Disability Benefits
If you have to give up work or go part-time the biggest pressure on you will be financial. There are a number of sickness and disability benefits that you may be eligible to claim; this can be a full time job in itself. If you have never claimed benefits before, the rules and regulations can seem specifically designed to put you off claiming. Do persevere. After all, this is one of the benefits you have contributed to throughout your working life with National Insurance payments. Do not think of yourself as

any less worthy of claiming just because you do not sit in a wheelchair or are not blind. You have a disability too. If that disability stops you from working you are entitled to some sort of benefit.

When you are ill, finding out about the benefits to which you are entitled can be another burden. Your local DHSS office or library will have leaflets explaining the benefits you can claim and we have included a brief guide here. The regulations may change from time to time so it is worth checking with your own DHSS office to find out if there have been any changes. The amounts you are able to claim change yearly so always check how much you are likely to get.

Statutory Sick Pay
If you are still working and earn enough to pay Class 1 National Insurance contributions you will usually get Statutory Sick Pay if you are off sick for four days or more. When you fall ill you should let your employer know straight away and send in a note from your doctor. You do not have to claim this benefit as your employer does it for you. Statutory Sick Pay is paid for up to 28 weeks in one period of sick leave.

If your employer stops paying you because he or she thinks you are fit for work you must ask for a reason and write to your social security office straight away. Send them any more sick notes and a detailed account of your illness. If the Department of Social Security asks you to return to work you can appeal against this decision. At this stage you would have to seek further advice from a welfare rights worker in your local council social services department.

Sickness Benefit
If your employer's obligation to pay Statutory Sick Pay runs out before 28 weeks is up, you may be able to claim Sickness Benefit. You can only claim Sickness Benefit if you have paid enough National Insurance contributions and are off sick for more than four days. Married women and widows who pay reduced rate National Insurance cannot claim Sickness Benefit unless they are claiming for an accident at work or an industrial disease.

Like Statutory Sick Pay, Sickness Benefit will be paid for up to 28 weeks. To claim it you should get form SSP1E or SSP1T from your employer if you are in work. Otherwise, you can get form SC1 from your social security office, doctor or hospital clinic.

If you have to go into hospital it is quite likely that some of your benefit will be stopped. The Social Security payments are calculated on the basis of your needs at home. It is assumed that when you go into hospital you will not be spending so much on food, heating and other bills so you do not need so much money. You are supposed to let your Social Security Office know the exact dates when you will be in hospital so that the payments can be revised. If you go into hospital and are allowed home for a few days before going back for further treatment do tell the DHSS as your benefits will be paid as normal for any time you are at home.

Invalidity Benefit
If you are still incapable of work when your Statutory Sick Pay or Sickness Benefit ends after 28 weeks you can claim Invalidity Benefit. You claim on the same form as the one used for claiming Sickness Benefit.

The Department of Social Security may decide, after an examination by one of their own doctors, that you are fit for work and no longer eligible for Invalidity Benefit. If this happens you can try and claim Unemployment Benefit or Supplementary Benefit and should sign on as unemployed with your local Social Security office. Not everyone will be eligible for these benefits, for instance if you are a married woman or cohabiting with someone who is employed, but it is always worth trying.

If the Department of Social Security does decide you are capable of work you should ask your doctor to keep sending in sick notes. The DHSS will then arrange for you to be examined by a second doctor. Benefit will only stop if this second doctor also deems you capable of work. If this happens you should take advice about an appeal against this decision and keep sending the sick notes to the DSS.

While you are waiting for the appeal, sign on as unemployed. This will not affect your right to appeal.

Severe Disablement Allowance
If you cannot get Sickness Benefit or Invalidity Benefit because you have not paid enough National Insurance contributions but you have been sick for 28 weeks or more, you may be eligible for Severe Disability Allowance. This payment is tax free, is not means tested and is available to men aged 16 to 64 and women aged 16 to 59. You may also be able to claim a payment for an adult dependent who may be a wife, a husband, or a person

looking after your child. You may also claim for each child that you have.

To claim this allowance use the form in leaflet NI 252 Severe Disablement Allowance available from your DSS. To claim, you must have been incapable of working through sickness for at least 28 weeks and be 80 per cent disabled. There are no hard and fast rules for deciding what is 80 per cent disabled. Your own doctor's reports will be used in the assessment and it is likely that you will be examined by a DSS appointed doctor who will assess each of your disabilities as a percentage and then add them up.

If the claim is unsuccessful you can appeal straight away. You should seek further advice if you need to do this.

Mobility Allowance
If you are unable or virtually unable to walk or have a degree of disability that makes it difficult or harmful to you to walk on your own more that a short distance, say 50 yards outside your house, this is the allowance to claim. It is really to help with the extra costs of transport, like taxi fares, that you might need.

It is difficult to predict which ME sufferers will qualify for this allowance. Doctors may not always appreciate that many sufferers are more mobile on some days than others. The best thing is to apply and see what happens. Apply on the form NI 211 Mobility Allowance from the DSS. You will probably be examined by a doctor and this examination will be arranged as near to your home as possible. If you find it difficult to get to the examination you can arrange to have the doctor visit you.

Attendance Allowance
After you have been ill for six months you can claim this payment if you need to be looked after by someone else. If you need help dressing and undressing, eating, washing and or going to the toilet you should claim this on the form in leaflet NI 205 Attendance Allowance.

This payment is independent of any National Insurance contributions you have made and is paid to you, not to the person looking after you. There are different levels of payment according to whether you need looking after during the daytime or during the day and at night. Once you have completed the form and sent it off, a doctor will visit you in your own home to make the assessment.

Invalid Care Allowance

This is the payment made to the person who looks after you. The carer will only be eligible if they spend at least 35 hours a week looking after someone who gets an Attendance Allowance. Use the form in leaflet NI 212 to claim this payment.

If you do not have enough money to live on, you may be able to claim Income Support. To claim this you, or your partner, must not work for more than 24 hours a week. And you must not have more than £6,000 in savings. If you pay rent or own a house you may also be able to get help with your rent or mortgage. To apply for both these benefits you should ask for an Income Support form at your Unemployment Benefit office or at the Post Office. A form for claiming housing benefit should also be included with this form.

Income Support payments include a personal allowance for yourself and a partner and an allowance for any child you look after, housing costs payments to cover some of the costs not met by housing benefit, and a premium payment. Premium payments are fixed payments for groups of people with special needs such as one parent families, or the disabled. Working out Income Support is complicated so ask your Social Security Office for advice. There are more details on leaflet SB20: A Guide to Income Support.

There are a number of other payments you may be able to claim in addition to these. You can claim back the cost of fares to and from hospital. If you need extra heating because you feel colder than most people you may be able to claim extra money. If you have been advised by your doctor to follow a special diet, or you need help with the cost of laundry bills, through incontinence, you may be able to get help.

ME sufferers have a certain disadvantage when making claims for disability payments because they often look perfectly normal, or at any rate look much better than they feel. It can be embarrassing discussing your problems with strangers so make sure your doctor has all the facts about the effect of ME on your life. You might like to ask him to write a full report including all your symptoms, the tests you have had, and the effect of ME on your physical capabilities.

You may find yourself minimising the effects of your illness if you are assessed on a good day. Make sure you tell the assessors exactly how ME has affected you and don't forget the wretched days when you have been confined to bed barely able to open your eyes through fatigue and pain. If you are nervous about being assessed you may like to have someone accompany you. This is perfectly acceptable. It may help to write down in advance some of the things you want to tell the assessing doctor.

It is hard to say whether the increasing publicity surrounding ME has made it any easier for sufferers to be believed by doctors. But at least they have almost certainly heard of the disease by now. Although it can be hard work claiming benefits it is well worth making the effort. You are unlikely to have as much money as you did when you were working , but at least you will not have the financial burden of no income at all.

11 Sex and Relationships

One of the most distressing things about ME is that it is not confined to one person. It has the capacity to destroy whole families – if you let it. The whole book has been aimed at helping you, the sufferer, to cope with ME. But your family may also need help in coping. While you may be grieving for the loss of your health, your family may be grieving for the loss of their once capable mother, their breadwinning father, their wife or husband. Grief is not too strong a word for the feelings that will occur in a family that is touched by ME. Children will grieve for the loss of a loving mother or father who once ran them to school, kicked a football around with them, took them on outings or just sat and talked. Your husband or wife will not only lose a capable partner who might have run the household while holding down a job, but they may have lost a lover.

The key to the whole family coping with ME is for them to find out as much about this illness as possible and for the other members of the family to try and understand what the sufferer is going through. This chapter has been written mainly for the family and friends of ME sufferers to help them cope with the changes in normal family life.

Your Partner
As the husband or wife of a sufferer you could be facing the biggest challenge of your life. The person you married may have changed from a lively, active person into someone who can barely stumble out of bed to the bathroom. In the early stages of ME your partner may sleep for 20 hours a day and you will probably feel that the person you married is little more than a zombie. If you had always shared the household chores you will find that it is up to you to make sure things run smoothly, putting an extra burden on you. In addition to this, your partner may suffer severe depression, mood swings, or just inappropriate behaviour. This can play havoc with your marriage unless you are strong enough to keep it going for both of you.

The most important thing any partner of an ME sufferer can do is to believe in their illness. This may be difficult. Many doctors still do not recognise ME as a disease. They may have told you that all it will take is a good night's sleep to get over it, or that it is all in the mind. If you are swayed by these views but your partner is convinced he or she is ill with ME, you should not automatically believe the doctors just because they are doctors and are supposed to know about these things. You can see with your own eyes that there is something drastically wrong with your partner. He or she needs all the help you can give them and the best way is to support them fully through this traumatic illness. If all you can say is 'pull yourself together' you are not only ruining your relationship but adding further suffering. Try and put yourself in their shoes. What would you be feeling if you were confined to the house, barely able to walk to the front door, let alone down the street? Would you want someone to tell you just to go and get a good night's rest?

As the partner of a sufferer you should make it your business to find out all you can about ME. The more you find out the more you will realise that ME is a real disease and is not something that is brought on by a severe bout of hypochondria. You cannot just 'shake off' ME like a bad cold. You may find it helpful to contact the ME Association or ME Action Campaign. Many partners or families of sufferers have joined the Association because there are particular problems in living with ME patients. You will probably find it good to talk to other people who have been in the same situation.

Practical Support

One of the most useful ways of supporting your partner is to accompany them on their visits to the doctor. ME sufferers often find it very difficult to concentrate and to remember exactly what the doctor is telling them. If you can visit at the same time and take notes of the details of medication, you will be giving your partner immeasurable support. If your partner has to make a journey to see the doctor he or she may be too tired when they arrive even to be able to explain what is wrong. You will be able to back up what your partner is saying, and give the doctor a better idea of the symptoms and how they are affecting the whole household. National health doctors have only a few minutes for each consultation, so you might find it helpful to make a list of symptoms and problems before the visit.

In previous years there were many anecdotal reports of marriages breaking up because one partner could not cope with the strain of living with an ME sufferer. In many cases this was because the partner could not accept that ME was a real disease and would not tolerate a spouse who could not pull him or herself together. If you cannot accept that ME is a real disease then your relationship is heading for disaster. You will not be able to give any of the support a sufferer needs and sooner or later something will give.

Once you have found out more about ME you will realise that you will have to take on much of the burden of running the household. You might find it too much that you are left with all the responsibilities of sorting out child care, shopping, bills, clean clothes, cooking, housework, DIY jobs and gardening, but until your partner is well enough to help out again you should be prepared to keep things running smoothly. This may mean extra work, it may be tiring, but you are lifting the burden of responsibility from your partner's shoulders so that he or she has the space to get better without worrying too much about everyday things. For an ME sufferer who has been used to running the household the worry of unpaid bills and lapsed housework can prove an unendurable stress.

Coping with changing moods
One thing that very few partners are prepared for is the change in mood a sufferer experiences during ME. If your partner had a sunny, happy personality it may come as a shock to find he or she has turned into a depressed, morose individual. This is where your support will be needed most.

Two common symptoms of ME are depression and anxiety. One of the most distressing things about depression is that the person suffering often does not realise that anything is wrong. It is up to the partner or family to look out for the warning signs of depression, for instance lack of interest in anything, loss of appetite, disturbed sleep. If you think your partner is depressed do not scold him or her for being unaffectionate or selfish; people with ME cannot help their moods or behaviour. Remember that depression is an illness. Do not tell them to pull themselves together. The ME sufferer will already be feeling guilty about his or her disease and the effect it has on the family. Your reproaches will only make it worse. Never underestimate the seriousness of depression because suicide is a risk, particularly if the person hints that they might be thinking of it. If they refuse to go to the doctor you would be wise to call the family doctor yourself.

Some sufferers find their mood changes swiftly from happy to sad and vice versa, or they find they cry at things that would not have bothered them before, for instance at a sharp remark. This is called emotional lability and is a common symptom of ME. You must be prepared for this, and if it happens, you must recognise it as part of the disease and not think your partner has undergone a permanent personality change.

Constant exhaustion and tiredness are very difficult to cope with. While you might want to go away for weekends, play tennis or invite friends round for dinner, all your partner might want to do is sleep. You will have to adapt to this new slower pace of life. Of course there is nothing stopping you going out with your friends but don't expect your partner to feel up to it all the time. You may have to learn to be more spontaneous and do things on the spur of the moment just because the sufferer is feeling energetic that day. If you do arrange an outing you must accept that your partner might have to spend the next day recovering from the exertion. You must come to recognise that when ME sufferers say they are tired they really mean it. They will find it difficult to carry on a conversation and may even feel too tired to sit and watch television for an evening. The tiredness of ME is not the sort that can be relieved by an hour's nap – it might mean having to go to bed for the rest of the day.

Entertaining friends or going out for the evening can be fraught with problems. The effort of getting ready to go out can prove too much for some sufferers and it can be disappointing if you have looked forward to doing something only to be thwarted by your partner's illness. One sufferer described how she spent an afternoon preparing for a dinner party and, although she had not cooked anything elaborate, the effort was too much and she had to sit like a zombie all evening without even the strength for conversation.

Your Sex Life

Sex is something that may also become problematic. You will come to realise that an ME sufferer becomes exhausted very quickly. They may have no energy left by the evening or they may feel the exertion is all too much. If your partner says they do not feel up to having sex then you must try and accept that – it

105

usually means they know they will be too tired to stay the course. However, sex is not completely out of the question with ME. You and your partner may have to adapt to having sex at those times of the day when the sufferer is feeling most energetic – this might be first thing in the morning or at lunchtime. Male sufferers report they sometimes have trouble in sustaining an erection although the urge to have sex is not diminished by ME. Once again, it is a case of fitting in sex when the urge is there. Although some sufferers find intercourse exhausting, many appreciate a massage or just hugging, kissing and stroking which, although not always so fulfilling, can be extremely pleasant. If you and your partner have been having some trouble communicating, one of the best ways to come back together and show each other you are still in love is by simple touching or massage or just lying quietly with each other.

Children
Many female ME sufferers have to make the decision of whether or not to start a family while they still have the illness. For some women, ME strikes during their most fertile years and many feel that if they do not take the plunge now they might miss out on the chance to have children. There have been no studies on ME and pregnancy. Some women report that their symptoms disappeared during pregnancy while some feel they got worse.

There is no evidence that babies of mothers with ME develop ME themselves. If you are worried about this you should talk it over with your doctor. Making the decision to have children is difficult at the best of times. As well as the questions of can we afford to have children, will we have to move house, can I keep on working, you will have to think about whether you can cope with a baby and ME. There are no hard and fast rules; you have to do what you think best. But you must be ready with back-up support if you have a relapse after the child is born. Remember, having a baby to look after is a 24-hour-a-day job and if there is just one hour of that day when you are too exhausted to move, you can bet that will be the time when your baby needs you most.

There is no doubt that when ME strikes at a member of the family everyone is affected. One woman who has had ME for more than ten years said: 'I don't feel bitter or resentful about having ME but I do sometimes feel pigsick at what it's done to my family. We've had to stay in the same house all the time because I couldn't do without my support network of family and friends.

My husband has had to turn down several offers to work abroad which would have boosted his career, because we've always had to be near someone who could look after the children if I was ill. We've had no choice in where to send the children to school. It's always had to be near enough for them to walk because I can't be relied upon to drive them.'

Everyone has to make sacrifices when ME comes into the family – this will either strengthen your relationship or break it. Only you can decide whether you are going to fight ME together or leave the sufferer to fight his or her own lonely battle.

The Single Sufferer
Being single with ME is no joke either. If you have no one living with you, you will not upset anyone else's routine but similarly you will have no one to help you in times of crisis. The single sufferer probably fights the loneliest battle against ME. If you have had to give up work you may become very cut off from the rest of the world and this can be dangerous. You should contact the ME Association who will put you in touch with other single ME patients, many of whom will have faced the same problems.

Many young people with ME have to move back to live with their parents. While they are lucky to have parents who will look after them it can sometimes be hard to move back to the home you once broke away from. One young woman who had been working in London before she came down with ME eight years ago said: 'I got what I thought was 'flu and went home to my parents to get over it. I haven't been well since. I felt dreadful about having to move back home because I saw it as a personal failure. My parents have been wonderfully supportive and they never expressed any doubt about my illness, but it was quite a relief to meet other people in the same boat through the ME Association. At first, I felt I was only staying temporarily with my parents. It's only the past year that I've accepted that I am living here and have got round to unpacking my books.'

Another problem with being a single ME sufferer is that you do not go out to meet other people of your own age or interests. There is a singles group that is part of the ME Association which is not so much a dating agency but more a means of meeting other single people of both sexes and making friends, even if it has to be done over the telephone.

Joining an evening class is often given as the ideal way of meeting a partner, but you should not just join a class or a club with the sole aim of meeting a mate. As luck would have it, generally the harder you try to attract someone as a partner the less successful you will be. It's as if you have a neon sign above your head wherever you go saying 'I'm desperate'. The best approach is to take it easy and play it cool. If you want to join an evening class or club, go ahead. But make sure you are doing it because it is something you genuinely want to do rather than just a means of finding your true love – the chances are he or she won't turn up.

If you do meet someone you like and want to have a relationship with, it can be difficult to tell them you have ME. With all the media attention that has been given to ME over the past few years few people will not have heard of it. What they might have heard is another matter. They might have read that it is Yuppie Flu, all in the mind, incurable or even infectious. They might have all sorts of preconceived ideas that would affect the way they react to a real-life ME sufferer.

Most other single ME sufferers would not advise you to plunge in straight away and tell them all about your illness. It would probably put most people off. Wait until you have seen the person you like a few times before giving them all the details. If they really like you and want to see more of you, something like ME should not put them off. If they turn rather cool you will know they are not the right person for you. But then, would you really want to go out with someone who cannot accept you as you are?

12 Sleep and Rest

One of the best ways of starting on the path to recovery for any ME sufferer is to recognise the need for proper rest. Right back at the start of the history of ME it was recognised that people who rested in the early stage of their illness recovered quicker than those who tried to carry on as normal. It may be very difficult to stop all your normal activities but, if you push yourself too much, you will only be harming your body still further.

You have to realise that your body has changed. It is not the same body that once jogged round the park every night. It is not the same body that slogged hard at work for 40 hours week. It is not the same body that battled through Sainsbury's on a busy Saturday morning. You have to get used to the idea that your capacity for exercise and even what you might have classed as normal activity has become drastically reduced. You must completely revise all your ideas about rest and inactivity. If you have always regarded excessive rest as a waste of time it will be very difficult to adjust, but, for your own sake, you must.

We are taught from a very early age that sleep is the great restorer. When we feel tired we sleep to regain enough energy for the next day. We count on a good night's sleep to make us fit for the next day and spend about one-third of our lives asleep. Most people do not give this much thought until their regular patterns of sleep are disturbed.

Sleep has two main functions: to restore energy levels and help the body synchronise itself into the regular rhythm of day and night. This may seem pretty obvious but there are some important chemical reactions that take place all night while you sleep and without them you cannot live.

If you deprive people of sleep for any length of time they start to hallucinate and show slightly psychotic behaviour. In addition to these behaviour changes, chemicals in the blood that carry energy to the cells are markedly depleted. When people are allowed to go to sleep after being deprived of sleep for several days these chemical imbalances sort themselves out and

109

behaviour returns to normal. There is something about being asleep that enables the body to restore these energy chemicals and it can only do it while you are asleep.

Sleep is also important in setting a biological rhythm that most other functions of the body fall in with. Temperature, pulse rate, and the production of certain chemicals in the brain all synchronise themselves with our own personal cycles of sleep and waking.

While most of the population would say that sleep was restful and restored their energy, most ME sufferers find that they sleep for many more hours than they used to and still wake up feeling tired. Sleep does not seem to perform its normal restorative function and to discover why this is you need to know more about sleep and what happens during sleep.

During the hours that you are asleep you will go through cycles of different types of sleep. As you drift off, your sleep gradually deepens until you are in a deep slumber but this does not last all night. Over about an hour-and-a-half you will return to a lighter sleep and then into a deeper sleep and back to light sleep. This sort of cycle lasts all night and each cycle lasts about an hour-and-a-half. As morning approaches each cycle becomes lighter and gradually things start happening to prepare your body for the morning – your body temperature rises, your pulse and breathing begin to speed up and levels of certain hormones begin to rise.

If you are woken during the deep sleep part of the cycle you will feel groggy, lethargic and irritable. If you wake during the light part of the cycle you will feel relatively wide awake, even if you have not had a whole night's sleep. That is because during the light cycle you are almost conscious anyway, so when you are woken you have not been dragged from the very depths of sleep. During these sleep cycles you are actually sleeping two types of sleep. Rapid Eye Movement (REM) sleep occurs during the light part of the cycle and is usually the time you dream. It is also called active sleep because you move around a lot and are restless. Non-Rapid Eye Movement (NREM) is the inactive sleep of the very deep slumber part of the sleep cycle.

REM sleep may be the most important part of the cycle as far as restoring lost energy is concerned. In experiments which have artificially deprived people of the REM portion of their sleep, it has been found that they make up for this loss in the nights after the deprivation by having longer REM parts of the cycle and shorter NREM parts of the cycle.

Not very much is known about hypersomnia, or too much sleep, which is a major complaint of ME sufferers. It is thought to be a disorder of the REM part of the sleep cycle. People with ME do not seem to have the right amount of REM sleep needed to replenish energy levels. To make up for this you have to sleep much more than the average person in order to catch up on your quota of REM sleep. It may be that your NREM cycles take over in some way from the REM cycles and you always feel groggy and tired when you wake up because you are always waking up during an NREM cycle.

No studies have been made of hypersomnia in ME but there are other diseases in which this symptom occurs such as liver failure, hypothyroidism (low thyroid function), diabetes, chronic lung disease, multiple sclerosis and viral encephalitis. In those cases the underlying disease can often be treated and this sorts out the excessive sleep. Narcolepsy, in which the primary symptom is excessive sleepiness during the day time is extremely rare. It is treated with drugs that stop the person nodding off and is believed to be due to a disorder of the REM part of the sleep cycle.

There is not very much that can be done for the ME sufferer who has hypersomnia. There are no drugs that will restore the REM part of the sleeping cycle. Some doctors would see hypersomnia as the body's way of building up enough energy, through sleep, to fight the chronic fatigue and the underlying persistent viral infection. There are some drugs that can be prescribed if you are prone to dropping off to sleep at odd times of the day but most doctors would tell you to sleep as much as you feel you need to – even if this is up to 18 hours a day.

Most ME sufferers gradually need less and less sleep as they start to recover from the disease. You may find you only need to rest for a couple of hours each afternoon to gather enough strength to carry on with the day. If you find that sleeping during the day makes you feel worse than ever you could try some sort of relaxation or meditation technique. This will allow you to relax totally without nodding off and some people find it is just as helpful as an hour's sleep. (Suitable techniques are described in Chapter 14 on alternative therapies.)

Living a life of constant sleep and rest can be very frustrating. You might feel that life is passing you by. Relatives and friends are getting on with their lives, making progress in their careers, marrying, having children, taking up new sports, going to the

111

theatre, taking holidays. It will be hard to cope with your own incapacity. What a normal person does in two weeks it might take you six months to achieve. But it is something you have to come to terms with. There is very little you can do to speed up the process of this illness; the only medicine is rest. If you try and cheat ME by plunging yourself into your former levels of activity you will only lose out and do yourself more harm than good.

The sooner you accept that and start resting, the sooner you will start to recover. And the odds are you will recover. It may take months, it may take years, but most sufferers do make something of a recovery, if not to full capacity again, at least to the levels of a person who can take life at a slow pace and find it enjoyable, rewarding and satisfying.

It might help you to look on this period of recovery as 'aggressive rest therapy'. Instead of lying back and accepting your illness you are fighting back with an active therapy. Your rest now has a purpose to it. Instead of lying around moping that you can no longer do things you want to, you can lie down thinking, 'this is the treatment I have prescribed and I must stick to it'.

Once you start to recover from ME, or feel able to potter about the house, you should not throw yourself into too much overactivity again. Obviously it is hard for anyone who has to look after children to be able to rest. It is often women with young children who take the longest to recover from ME because much of their energy is spent in caring for their needs. If you are in this position you must start caring for your own needs too – you must embark on a programme of aggressive rest therapy straight away.

One woman who has had ME for more than ten years contracted the disease when her two children were aged just nine months and two. She had to relinquish their care to her mother and a very close friend who lived nearby. 'When I first had ME I felt very resentful. I couldn't play with my children or even feed them. I was so weak I couldn't even feed myself.'

If you have someone to whom you can pass on the responsibility of caring for your children, you are very lucky and can devote all your energy to rest and recovery. It is more likely that you will have to shoulder these responsibilites yourself. In that case you must try and conserve as much energy as possible and rest as much as you can. You will have to stop worrying about little day-to-day things like whether the sheets need ironing or the floor needs vacuuming. You will have to change your way of thinking. Instead of saying 'I have to go to the shops' you must say 'do I have to go to the shops?' If it is not absolutely necessary to exert yourself, then don't. Follow the maxim 'Don't stand when you can sit and don't sit when you can lie down'.

You must try and think of ways of avoiding strenuous work so that you can have time for yourself. If you are extremely disabled you may be able to get help with cleaning through your social services department. If not, you might think about investing in a cleaner for a few hours a week. If you find shopping difficult there may be a firm near you that delivers. Cut down on ironing by skipping out the sheets. In winter, when shirts are covered by jumpers, iron only the collars and cuffs or pay other people to iron them for you. Of course paying for these services could become expensive but you have to ask yourself 'Isn't it worth it to regain my health?'

Sleep and rest are now available on the NHS. London's Charing Cross Hospital has treated more than 20 ME patients. Although they think ME may be caused by the effects of overbreathing the Charing Cross team use the same approach to trying to cure ME – rest and relaxation – as they do with patients recovering from a heart attack. The team, led by cardiologist Dr Peter Nixon, believe that ME may be caused by hyperventilation or over-breathing. The theory was developed after studying heart disease patients, almost all of whom hyperventilate. (The principles of hyperventilation have been explained in Chapter 5.) To recap, if you start hyperventilating, the balance of oxygen and carbon dioxide in the blood is shifted, changing the acidity of the blood. This imbalance means that normal chemical reactions in the body cannot take place because the conditions are not quite right. This upsets the whole body and leads to a range of symptoms including fatigue, sleep problems, headaches, inability to concentrate, bowel disorders and blurred vision.

Some ME patients attending Dr Nixon's clinic are 'put to sleep' with drugs for days at a time to help sort out the breathing disorder. Since respiration is one of the body functions that is regulated by sleep, it is not surprising that this forms part of the treatment and many people are said to be helped by it. The treatment teaches people how to control their breathing so that they do not hyperventilate and to recognise the warning signs or situations that might lead them to overbreathe.

One London housewife who had suffered with ME for more

than two years said of Dr Nixon's treatment: 'They offered me the one thing I had really wanted from the very beginning – the chance to have a total rest. Then they started teaching me to breathe properly, and I gradually began to get my mind back again, to be able to think.' She is now recovering both mentally and physically from her illness. 'My body is still somewhat clapped out after a year of inaction, and it will take some months to get it back into some sort of working order. But I am going out for walks, for swims, to church, whereas before I couldn't walk the length of our garden without ending up in bed.'

It is often quite difficult to tell if you are hyperventilating as the movement of the chest may be very subtle. A simple way to find out is to put one hand on the upper chest and the other on the upper tummy. Only the hand on your tummy should move. If you feel you are overbreathing and you want to stop it there is a simple exercise you can do.

Lie down on the floor on your stomach with arms outstretched, elbows bent and hands crossed beneath your forehead. Breathe gently until you feel comfortable and relaxed. Concentrate on the breath entering your body. Imagine it is a column that fills your chest and abdomen. If you are breathing properly you should feel your stomach swell out like a balloon beneath you as you press against the floor. Spend five or ten minutes doing this and really relaxing and then slowly get up. You should be able to breathe properly without thinking about it. If you notice that your breathing pattern has gone awry get back on the floor and try again.

If you find that you cannot breathe properly you should ask your doctor for help. While breathing properly may not actually cure your ME, it will help to relieve many superfluous symptoms that may have developed over the years.

Plenty of sleep, rest, relaxation and deep breathing sound too easy to be the cure for a disease as devastating as ME, but all of them will help you feel better.

13 Treatment from Doctors: anti-viral drugs, anti-depressants and EPD

At the moment there is no cure for ME. There is no drug that a doctor can prescribe that will cure the underlying disease although there are a number of drugs you might be given to relieve some of its symptoms.

When you first visit your doctor you will probably be subjected to many tests. These are not tests to diagnose ME but tests to exclude other diseases that have similar symptoms. For instance, hypothyroidism, a disease which stops the thyroid gland producing enough hormone, has symptoms in common with ME – low body temperature, poor concentration and fatigue.

Anaemia, Addison's disease, hypothyroidism, multiple sclerosis, some cancers, AIDS, deficiencies of some minerals and tuberculosis are all associated with profound fatigue. All these can be excluded with blood tests. If you are certain you suffer from ME it can be frustrating having a battery of tests conducted and probably getting consistently negative results, but be patient. Your doctor is only trying to help by excluding every possibility before making the diagnosis of a disease that has no easy cure or a definite outcome.

Because there is no definitive test for ME your doctor should make a clinical diagnosis based on the type of symptoms you have and the length of time you have had them. A test developed at St Mary's Hospital in London will reveal if you have raised antibody levels to enteroviruses but only around half of the ME sufferers have these raised levels. Some have abnormal ratios of the T-helper cells and T-suppressor cells that are involved in the immune response. But this is not true of all sufferers. While abnormal results might be comforting for you and your doctor – proving there really is something wrong – they are not essential for the diagnosis. Until better tests have been developed, no ME patient should rely on a test for a diagnosis. Your clinical symptoms will indicate to the doctor if you really have ME.

Diagnosing ME can be fraught with difficulty but curing it is even more of a problem. There are several drugs that might help some of your symptoms. Analgesics might relieve muscle and joint pain and anti-depressants might lift your mood, relieve insomnia and help restore sleeping patterns to normal. This symptom relief is something that only you and your doctor can sort out.

However, there are some drugs and treatments that seem to be useful in treating ME in some people. And there are new lines of research that could be the key to a cure.

Anti-Viral Drugs and Immunostimulants
When a virus enters the body the different white blood cells, or lymphocytes, that form part of the immune system are stimulated to mount a defence. There are several types of lymphocyte which initiate the attack on a virus, maintain that attack until all the virus is killed and then suppress the attack when the job is done. Some lymphocytes will do this by producing an antibody or a toxic chemical that will kill the virus. Others have the ability to recognise a specific virus and then kill it. The cells controlling this immune response are the T-helper lymphocytes.

In ME these T-helper lymphocytes appear to bear the brunt of the damage wreaked by the virus. The T-cell lymphocytes do not seem to recognise that the virus is a danger and do not initiate the normal immune response. The virus may use the genetic material of the T-cell lymphocyte to produce its daughter viruses. Some of the T-cell lymphocytes may then die or fail to function properly and the rest of the lymphocytes involved in the immune response get out of synch – they cannot respond properly to infections.

If ME is caused by a persistent viral infection and a damaged immune response, theoretically it should be possible to develop a cure that would remove the virus and/or stimulate the flagging immune system to fight the virus.

Anti-Viral Drugs
There are a number of anti-viral drugs on the market but so far they have not been very effective in the treatment of ME. Many of them are specific to one type of virus, for instance acyclovir is used to treat Herpes virus infections like shingles. These drugs will not kill off a wide range of viruses; unlike an antibiotic which

will work against several different bacteria, anti-virals only work against one type of virus.

None of the anti-viral drugs available act specifically against the enteroviruses that are thought to be important in ME. In many ME patients there are no antibodies to show which virus caused the illness and no evidence of a persistent virus infection, so anti-viral drugs will probably be no help. In addition, these anti-viral therapies appear to be more effective in the acute stage of the illness. A diagnosis of ME will not be made until you have been ill for at least six months, or have failed to recover from the infection. By that time the virus may no longer be present in your body in its virulent form so there is no point taking an anti-viral drug.

However there is one exception. A handful of ME patients claim to have been helped by an anti-viral drug called amantadine (brand name Symmetrel), that is more commonly used to treat Parkinson's disease.

Amantadine was first developed as an anti-influenza drug and is still used to prevent cases of Asian 'flu in groups such as the elderly and heart patients who would succumb very easily to a bad bout of 'flu. Amantadine was discovered as a drug for Parkinson's disease in the late 1960s when it markedly reduced the symptoms in a patient given the drug to fight influenza. Since then its use as an anti-viral has largely been overlooked.

Christopher Monckton, a journalist on London's *Evening Standard*, says his remarkable recovery from ME was due solely to the use of amantadine. Monckton suffered from ME for two years between 1983 and 1985 and had been forced to give up his job as policy advisor to the Prime Minister because of his illness. His GP told him: 'I'm not going to be beaten by this. I'm determined to find the answer.' After a fortnight of telephone calls to medical colleagues Monckton's GP came up with an answer – amantadine. After just five days of treatment Monckton says he was cured. He says: 'Two years of miserable illness came to an end. I woke up feeling well.'

Monkton's GP has had success in treating other ME patients with amantadine, but he says that the people who seem to do the best are ME patients whose symptoms are mostly cerebral. The success rate is poor in patients whose major symptoms are physical.

Unfortunately the evidence for amantadine is purely anecdotal. We cannot advise its use at the moment as side-effects have been reported.

Immunostimulants

Several approaches have been taken in trying to repair the damaged immune system with drugs that might act as immuno-stimulants.

Gammaglobulin: One approach that was tried in the mid-1980s was the use of injections of gammaglobulin to give patients the antibodies they would need to fight a virus. Gammaglobulin is a plasma product derived from the blood of hundreds of people who have had a viral infection. It contains antibodies to all the viruses that are thought to cause ME and is given as an injection. It was hoped that by giving patients the antibodies they seemed to lack they would be able to fight off the infection. Although some patients seemed to improve, the results were not consistent and the injections sometimes made the patient feel worse; it was not possible to predict which patients would improve.

Transfer Factor: A similar approach that has largely been discredited by the orthodox medical profession is the use of injections of transfer factor. This treatment is used by just a handful of doctors in Britain, mainly specialists in treating food and chemical allergies. Transfer factor is thought to be a chemical that is secreted by white blood cells when they are stimulated to fight infections. It is derived from the blood of people who have successfully fought viral infections in the past. Despite intensive investigations no one knows what transfer factor actually is – it is such a small molecule that it is very difficult to isolate in a test tube. It has been suggested that it is genetic material that works by supplying the patient with the correct genetic code for making antibodies.

Injections of transfer factor are thought to teach the damaged immune system what to do. White blood cells that do not recognise a virus are 'taught' how to recognise one again and hopefully to destroy it.

Although there have been no scientific studies of transfer factor in ME sufferers, some people claim to have been helped by it. In the mid-1970s it was hailed as a cure for multiple sclerosis but extensive clinical trials failed to show any improvement whatsoever. One of the things that suggests it does not work is the size of the molecule. Transfer factor is so small it is unlikely to be able to do physically what it is supposed to do.

Anti-depressants

While anti-depressants are often prescribed to ME sufferers to treat their depression (as discussed in Chapter 9), those tricyclics which have sedative properties can greatly improve sleeping habits. For many ME sufferers, and their families, the most difficult problems to deal with are sleeping disorders. You might be awake all night while the rest of the household is asleep and then sleep all day. You may find you sleep for up to 20 hours a day but still wake up feeling tired.

While these problems are often caused by food allergies (for instance an allergy to wheat might produce a 'high' that makes sleep impossible for several hours) there is one simple thing you can do first to try and sort them out without resorting to drugs and before getting into the complexities of dealing with food allergies. If you have problems getting to sleep at night you should think about the foods and drinks you are taking in the afternoon and evening. If you are drinking tea, coffee, cocoa and caffeine-laden fizzy drinks during the day, try and cut down as it may be you are filling yourself up with excessive amounts of stimulants like caffeine and theobromine that will still be in your system when you go to bed and will stop you sleeping.

It may sound remarkably simplistic to tell you to watch what you are eating and drinking. Most people know that caffeine is a stimulant that prevents sleep; what many people do not realise is that caffeine may linger in the body for a few hours after you have had that cup of tea or coffee. And the length of time caffeine stays in the body varies from person to person. If you are particularly sensitive to caffeine you may find that cutting it out during the afternoon and evening will help you to sleep better at night.

It may be tempting to drink alcohol during the evening as it does make you feel sleepy. However, later on in the night your sleep will be disturbed as an effect of the alcohol, and you will not feel rested in the morning. So try to avoid it. Alcohol also has other effects on ME sufferers so it is wise to cut it out altogether (see Chapter 6).

If you are sleeping during the day and finding it difficult to sleep at night, ask yourself whether you really need those day-time naps. You may actually be getting all the sleep you need but not at the times you want it. You may find it helpful to rearrange your sleeping times. If you have great difficulty in sleeping, for instance you wake up very early or you sleep for many hours without feeling rested, anti-depressants could be helpful. Of course it is impossible for us to say whether every ME sufferer would benefit; it is something you must talk over with your doctor.

One of the symptoms of depression is very early waking and not being able to get back to sleep. Of course it is not the only symptom of depression and your doctor is unlikely to make a diagnosis of depression solely on the basis of your sleeping habits. Very often the tricyclic anti-depressants which also have sedative properties will help to regulate sleep and lift your mood at the same time. Don't feel bad if your doctor prescribes anti-depressants. You may not have realised how low your mood was and your doctor is not writing you off as a psychiatric case; he or she is just trying to help you over some of your immediate problems, one of which may be a sleep disorder.

The tricyclics work by modifying the levels of certain chemicals in the brain that are responsible for your mood and sleep mechanisms. Some of these chemicals are also found outside the brain so the drug may cause side-effects like dry mouth, blurred vision, constipation, dizziness and drowsiness. Not everyone suffers from side-effects, but if you have any of these problems that are not the symptoms you had as a result of your ME, you should tell your doctor. Usually, the side-effects pass within a fortnight and it may be worth sticking it out.

Sometimes you may have side-effects but the drug does not seem to be working. This is because the drug will usually take a few days, sometimes up to two weeks, to have an effect, so don't give up. Even if your sleep problems clear up within a few weeks your doctor will tell you to carry on taking the tablets for a few months.

One drug that seems to help some sufferers is a tricyclic anti-depressant called dothiepin (brand name Prothiaden). It helped Nicky Spurgeon, whose case history is reported in chapter 16, and it helped one New Zealand sufferer to return to normal life after nearly 20 years of battling with ME. She said in *Meeting Place*, the journal of the Australian and New Zealand ME Society: 'Sudden attacks of exhaustion seemed to strike without warning . . . I would crawl to the nearest bed or sofa, lying there in a semi-stupor, cold and helpless until a little strength returned to my muscles and I could shuffle off for a hottie or a cup of tea. I became a vehicle without a petrol gauge, never knowing when I'd run out of gas and without any idea how long it would be before my tank was replenished enough to undertake another run.'

After years of trying different therapies this sufferer, Elizabeth, returned in desperation to her GP. 'I can't recall how many days I rested to travel the 24 miles to my GP. I do recall, however, my feeling of utter despair when told the medication he wished to prescribe was an anti-depressant.'

Her dosage started at 25 milligrams a day, rising daily to a maximum of 150 milligrams taken each night one-and-a-half hours before going to bed. She was told to telephone her doctor every day to give a progress report.

'Whatever dire things I expected to happen failed to materialise. I suffered nothing worse than some nausea, slight woosiness, a very dry mouth and initially no improvement. There was no noticeable improvement for at least a month to six weeks. Gradually, however, my appetite increased and sleep became sound. Energy levels rose gradually and an awareness that everyday chores previously resulting in exhaustion were now completed with relative ease. I began to wake each morning feeling rested, a forgotten feeling. Hope returned that I might again manage to play golf, drive the car a reasonable distance, have my grandchildren to stay or have friends for a weekend without total exhaustion being the price to pay for such innocent enjoyment.'

For the first time in ten years Elizabeth managed to work full-time – at a kiwi fruit packing-house – before succumbing to a passing 'flu virus that took several weeks to get over. Now retired, she lives a virtually normal life while recognising her limitations.

'It is clear that Prothiaden is no cure,' she said. 'Life before Prothiaden was one of total unpredictability. I don't know where I go from here. I certainly dislike intensely having to rely on this or any other medication to maintain the normal routine of daily living. I think though that I have become reasonably pragmatic and now consider the quality of life more important than its purity.'

The GP who recommended Prothiaden said he believed the drug was aiding recovery by inducing a more restful and energy-restoring type of sleep and that other anti-depressants without this sedative effect were not so helpful.

Many ME sufferers might be loath to take a drug that is so closely associated with psychological problems. It is worth noting that tricyclics were first developed for the treatment of hayfever before it was discovered that they lifted mood more effectively than they helped the hayfever. So they came to be called tricyclic anti-depressants and were used to help depression. They have been used for about twenty years now to help patients to sleep more soundly. Often patients also stop losing weight and they find that some of their brain fag is lifted and they can think more clearly. If you are not prepared to at least try this therapy you will never know if you might have been helped by it.

But one problem with just accepting a drug that is doled out by your doctor is that it makes you less motivated to learn about your illness. We would say that anyone who tries an anti-depressant should also be learning about their illness and finding out if Candida or food allergies are also a problem. The approach to ME should be an holistic one. You should avoid regarding drugs as magic bullets that will effect an immediate cure – there is no such 'cure' for ME. Drugs like Prothiaden may help relieve the symptom of disordered sleep but they will do nothing about the cause.

Enzyme Potentiated Desensitisation
If your doctor suspects you are suffering from food intolerance or allergies he or she may prescribe a course of injections called EPD or enzyme potentiated desensitisation. EPD was developed more that 20 years ago by Dr Len McEwen while working at St Mary's Hospital in London. It consists of injections of a solution of foods and inhalants to which you would be most likely to be allergic. Included in the solution are enzymes which increase the effect of the injections (hence 'enzyme potenti-ated'). Rather like a vaccination, EPD is thought to stimulate the immune system into producing antibodies against the allergen. Your immune system 'gets used' to dealing with the substances in the injection so that when you next eat an allergenic food your reaction will be far less severe, if there is any reaction at all.

Dr Michael Jenkins at the Royal London Homeopathic Hospital uses EPD in some of his ME patients if food allergy is suspected. Injections of EPD are given every two months to keep the patient 'topped up'. Patients are instructed to go on a very strict diet starting 24 hours before the injection and lasting until 48 hours afterwards. The diet normally consists of lamb and potatoes or pork and carrots and the aim is to exclude all possible allergenic foods during the time of the injection. If you take vitamin C or evening primrose oil supplements you will be advised to discontinue them for two weeks before and after an injection.

The injection normally makes people feel quite ill for a day and it takes several sessions to reach full effect. It often takes at least four injections before ME patients start to improve. But Dr McEwen, now in private practice, cites the case of one patient who tried to commit suicide 33 times. Since 1982, when she first met Dr McEwen, she has had an EPD injection every three months and has slowly improved.

Only three NHS doctors have any great experience of EPD and use it regularly: Dr Jenkins at the Royal Homeopathic Hospital, Dr Norman Williamson, area immunologist for the North-west health authority, and Dr Alan Franklin, a paediatrician in Chelmsford, Essex. It is a fairly costly course of treatment and most NHS hospital budgets will not run to the expense.

Angela, whose case history is given at the beginning of this book, says: 'To be honest I did not think EPD would make much difference. But Dr Jenkins said that as well as helping me with food allergies it would help me cope better with the chemicals that were a problem for me. It took four injections at two-monthly intervals before I noticed any difference but then I began to improve considerably. But it wasn't all plain sailing. I was very badly affected by the first three injections and I was having homeopathic drops at the same time, all of which upset me and made me feel worse.

'I had very bad migrainous headaches and I also had vomiting and diarrhoea. One of the homeopathic dilutions was of Coxsackie virus. I had a very bad response to that and was terribly ill. I was an in-patient at the Royal Homeopathic Hospital for four days and the doctor insisted that I had a room to myself, otherwise I might be affected by the other patients' deodorants, hair sprays and perfumes.'

Angela has had eight injections now, as has a close friend of hers who also has ME, and both are continuing to improve. They are not the only ones. It seems that many ME sufferers do develop food allergies and EPD has one major advantage over other methods of controlling food allergies, such as elimination diets and desensitising drops or injections: it requires little effort on behalf of the patient. In fact, it could almost be called the lazy patient's way of allergy control. Instead of spending much time and effort playing detective, the sufferer simply presents him or herself for injection.

But EPD is not a miracle cure, there are some drawbacks. First the sufferer must be patient. There will probably be no improvement for at least six months. Secondly, EPD will not deal with chemical allergies – although the fact that the patient will react less to allergenic foods can only help to strengthen the immune system and make the patient more tolerant of problem chemicals. Thirdly, there are some foods that EPD just will not desensitise the patient against; these are chicken, raw apples, raw carrots and celery.

At first sight, EPD may seem to be irrelevant in the case of ME, an illness that appears to be caused by chronic viral infection. But Dr McEwen says: 'The likely explanation is that the constant but inadequate immunological response to a virus that is never eliminated stimulates and deregulates the immune system in other directions.'

14 Treatment: alternative therapies

Anyone trying to find help from an alternative medical practitioner might find themselves slightly fazed by the range that is
available. You might have heard of acupuncture, homeopathy,
osteopathy, herbalism, hypnotherapy, but what about colour
therapy, reflexology, iridology or psionic medicine? Just the
names of these therapies can be a bit daunting. What do they all
mean and what do they do?

It is possible that all these techniques have been used at some
time to help people with ME with varying degrees of success. But
in this chapter we are going to limit our discussion to the
complementary therapies that seem to help the majority of ME
patients who try them.

When you first visit a complementary practitioner you will find
it very different from going to your GP. The most noticeable
difference is that the practitioner will spend most of the first
consultation finding out about you, your health and other aspects
of your life. It may take more than an hour to complete this case
history but few practitioners would commence treatment
without it. It may also be of some value to you in having someone
new to talk to about your ill health.

You should not expect any treatment to work immediately.
Some therapies, like acupuncture, take several sessions to start
having an effect – if they are going to have one at all. It is
impossible to say how quickly a treatment will work as so much
depends on you and your particular health problems.

Homeopathy
This philosophy on which homeopathy is based regards all
organisms as in a state of constant repair with considerable
capacity for overcoming the cause of any disease if you can
stimulate that capacity. The success of a cure depends on each
patient. Homeopaths believe there are no incurable diseases,
only incurable patients – the symptoms are not from the disease

but they are merely an expression of the body in its reaction to the underlying problems.

Diagnosis normally involves asking the patient what changes from normal health he or she has experienced including physical, emotional and sensory changes. You may be quite surprised at the depth of questioning when you first visit a homeopath. You may tell the practitioner about your aches and pains and the practitioner will ask what time of day they occur, whether the pain is continuous or fluctuates throughout the day. You might be asked how you are affected by different weather conditions or changes in temperature. You will be asked about your moods and emotions so that the practitioner can build up a psychological as well as physical profile of you.

Names of diseases are not used in homeopathy but your symptoms will be defined by the treatment that is used. Some of the treatments are not so dissimilar to those used by conventional medicine. Some of the live vaccines used in orthodox medicine to protect you against certain viruses are in fact highly diluted solutions of the virus; they stimulate your immune system to make antibodies that will defend your body against future infection without producing the disease itself. Homeopaths may use plant, mineral and sometimes animal materials to formulate their remedies. Occasionally a remedy may even be formulated from the pathogen that is thought to cause the symptoms, for instance Coxsackie virus or one of the influenza viruses.

There is a great deal of controversy about how homeopathic remedies work. Most are so diluted that it is almost beyond belief that any of the original material could still be present. Some American and French physicists have put forward the theory that rather than there being a chemical of the original substance left in the dilution, the original chemical leaves an imprint of itself on the water molecules when they are shaken together. The water molecules 'remember' what the original chemical was. They then act as a sort of template to tell water molecules in the body what the original chemical was. So these remedies are not chemicals but information about chemicals. This all sounds far-fetched but no more plausible theory has been found to explain how homeopathic remedies could possibly work. However, not all homeopaths use such diluted materials; many of them use remedies of a higher potency depending on the individual patient.

One doctor who sees NHS patients referred by their GPs is Dr

Jenkins who runs the outpatient clinic at the Royal London Homeopathic Hospital. He specialises in illnesses that have an allergy connection including asthma, arthritis, irritable bowel syndrome, migraine and, increasingly over the last two years, ME. Like all homoeopaths he takes a long case-history. Some patients will have their sweat analysed to see if they are deficient in any minerals. Sweat analysis is thought to be a more accurate way to test for certain mineral deficiencies than analysis of hair or blood. Most of the patients with ME that he has treated are deficient in zinc and magnesium and for these supplements are prescribed. If candidiasis is suspected Dr Jenkins prescribes nystatin, vitamin and mineral supplements and helps patients embark on an anti-Candida diet.

Dr Jenkins says ME patients tend to fall into two categories. These are those who have a clear history of good health until they were struck down with a 'flu-like illness followed by post-viral syndrome. The others cannot pinpoint the start of their illness to a particular viral infection but instead report a slow decline in health and have symptoms which suggest candidiasis or food intolerance. Many of the patients with food intolerance are treated with EPD (see Chapter 13). If Dr Jenkins suspects a persistent viral infection he may try homeopathic dilutions of the virus to stimulate the patient's immune system into fighting the infection.

There have been very few clinical trials to compare homeopathic remedies with more conventional medicines but there is some evidence that the body can be stimulated to heal itself. For instance, animal cells poisoned with arsenic and then given homeopathic doses of the same poison will recover and start to grow again.

Relaxation Techniques
Almost 50 years ago Dr Hans Selye showed that animals under experimental stress conditions developed physical diseases like heart disease, indigestion, gastric ulcers and a disturbed immune system. Today it is widely accepted that stress or anxiety can undermine the immune system and therefore lower resistance to almost any disease. Most diseases seem to have some sort of psychological as well as physical and environmental dimension and ME is no exception.

Everyone, sick or healthy, can benefit from the wide range of relaxation techniques that are now available. Yoga, meditation, hypnotherapy, biofeedback, concentrative breathing exercises (described in Chapter 12), massage, autogenic training and stress management courses can all be used to teach you how to relax. You must find the one that suits you.

Transcendental Meditation

One ME sufferer who has been greatly helped by transcendental meditation is Brenda Boisson. She had suffered from ME for two-and-a-half years before she read about the disease in a newspaper and recognised her symptoms. Her GP referred her to Dr William Weir, consultant immunologist at London's Royal Free Hospital. She saw him once a month for four months and went through a range of blood tests. Dr Weir recognised that one of Brenda's major problems was stress – she just could not relax. He said that if she did not learn how to relax it would prevent her recovering from ME. He advised her to contact the Transcendental Meditation Centre in Chelmsford, not far from where she lived, to find out about relaxation. After attending two talks at the Centre Brenda signed up for a four-day meditation course and she has never looked back. After only a week Brenda says she felt better and now, eight months later, she says she feels about 80 per cent better. She now meditates for at least 40 minutes a day, 20 minutes in the morning and evening.

'I was very ill. I could only walk about 100 yards at the most, I had to really struggle to get upstairs. I could hardly hang out the washing my arm ached so much. I had terrible pains in my arms and legs and felt so incredibly exhausted I spent most of the day lying down. I would get up and try to prepare a meal but even peeling potatoes was too much for me and I would have to go and lie down again.

'I know I was under a lot of stress and I think that is what TM has done for me – removed most of the stress. My muscles, particularly those in my back, were incredibly knotted and as soon as I started doing TM the tension just fell away and the muscles were much better.'

Brenda has improved so much she only sees Dr Weir once every six months and she is confident she will continue to improve.

Relaxing is surprisingly difficult for people who are not used to it; just lying down is not enough, your mind has to relax as much as your body. There are many different relaxation courses available. Generally you will be in a calm environment with nothing harsh around you like fluorescent lights for instance. As a trainee you will be helped into a comfortable posture, such as lying like a corpse on the floor with hands upwards. The teacher will give you instructions and help you to relax parts of the body in turn, and once you are completely relaxed you will be encouraged to let your mind go. You may be told to concentrate on your breathing or listen to a piece of music.

Relaxation techniques have been used to help asthmatics, patients undergoing cancer therapy, in pain relief, to lower high blood pressure and to control anxiety. So there is no reason why ME patients should not benefit from something that is so simple.

Biofeedback

Biofeedback is particularly useful in teaching people how to control stress-related conditions. Machines used to monitor muscle tension or breathing can be used as a graphic measurement of how stress affects you. A needle on a dial indicates your normal relaxed muscle state and if you go into tension the needle will move. Gradually you are taught how to control the movement of the needle, by relaxing, so that you can deal with your own stress. Biofeedback is sometimes available on the NHS and is used widely in pain relief clinics to help patients relax and avoid migraines or headaches.

Self-hypnosis

Self-hypnosis is also widely used to help relaxation. People in a hypnotic state become very relaxed and in the 1930s it was realised that people could relieve their own stresses through self-hypnosis. You are not in a trance but in a deep state of relaxation and the idea is that this relaxed state will carry you through your normal life. Hypnotherapy is another technique that is used in NHS pain clinics to relieve muscle aches and pains. It is also used to help cancer victims through the terminal stages of their illness and is even used in childbirth to help relieve pain.

Visualisation

Some relaxation techniques try to get you to fight your illness. Visualisation techniques will encourage you to develop a positive mental attitude towards life and to 'visualise' that you are getting well. The idea is that you imagine your immune system fighting and defeating this invading virus to help beat the infection.

Autogenic Training

Dr Kai Kermani is a full-time GP and trained psychotherapist who runs courses in Autogenic Training, a powerful technique for inducing deep relaxation. He encourages trainees to get in touch with their emotions, to off-load negative feelings and to come to feel and trust their personal strength and power to fight back.

Dr Kermani believes that by strengthening the mind in every possible way and helping a person to get out and truly live again, the body is made stronger and can benefit from orthodox medicine.

Massage

Every ME sufferer should consider massage, which is a considerably undervalued technique of healing. Most sufferers cannot take any form of exercise so the muscles gradually waste away and the blood circulation becomes very sluggish. This is not healthy. However ill you are, you need to keep your muscular tone and blood circulation as normal as possible – massage is one of the easiest ways of doing it.

Massage works on the muscles and ligaments of the body but its benefits go much further than that in keeping nerves and the blood system functioning normally. Massage will ease the tensions and knotted tissue in the muscles, increase the circulation of the blood and stimulate the lymphatic system, helping to get rid of waste materials from the body.

There are several types of massage but the most commonly used is based on Swedish techniques with four basic movements. Effleurage is a stroking movement that is meant to soothe you by relaxing the muscles in preparation for stronger movements. Pettrisage involves kneading, rolling and squeezing the tissues. Friction is small circular movement against the bone designed to relieve specific areas of tension. Tapotement is the hacking and flicking movements of the hands to stimulate, tone and strengthen the muscles. A massage session is usually ended with a few minutes of more effleurage movements.

Many masseurs will use aromatherapy oils in conjunction with a massage. Peppermint oil will help to relieve muscle pain and stimulate the blood flow while basil is said to lift your mood.

Of course you need not got to a professional for a massage and there are many shops now which stock massage and aromatherapy oils. Your partner may be the ideal masseur – on hand whenever you need him or her. Massage is more than a muscle stimulant it also fulfils a basic human need for bodily contact. Touch is vitally important in our day-to-day lives. American researchers have conducted experiments in which people were deprived of human body contact for days at a time. The subjects reported feeling painfully isolated, anxious and cut off from other people. We may not always be aware of it but touch is a basic human instinct to show our feelings and to demonstrate to others that they are loved. If ME has been coming between you and your partner a massage session may be just the thing to help you show each other that you really do need each other.

There are some situations, however, where massage should not be attempted. If you are in the acute inflammatory stage of arthritis, have a fever or other sort of inflammation you should wait until these have subsided before trying massage. If you have an infectious skin condition it is unwise to have a massage – you risk spreading the disease to other parts of your body and your masseur.

Massage has so many benefits that every ME sufferer should make sure there is a part of their day devoted to it. Your muscles will be in a stronger position to recover from your illness and massage will help relieve any stresses that may have built up during the day. Your local health food shop may be the best place to find someone who gives a really good massage. Qualified masseurs, many of whom have a very intuitive healing ability, often put their cards on health shop notice boards.

Colonics
One of the most interesting theories to explain the continuing ill health of ME sufferers is the concept of the 'toxic colon'. It is thought that wastes, hostile bacteria and viruses that build up in the colon may be responsible for many ME-like symptoms which can make your ME seem much worse than it really is. Some people even believe it is the cause of ME. Enteroviruses – the viruses that are believed to cause ME – live in the colon. An hypothesis put forward by the ME Action Campaign to explain the condition suggests that the presence of these viruses in the colon produces all the symptoms of the illness.

The colon is basically five feet of tubing at the end of your digestive system. It runs up the right hand side of your body, across just under the ribcage and down to the rectum. Its main function is to remove water and any nutrients left in the digested food after it has passed through the duodenum and ileum. As in the rest of the digestive system the colon is colonised by a variety of bacteria. In the main these are beneficial bacteria called Lactobacillus that help to digest our foods but there are also some harmful bacteria that are normally kept in check by Lactobacillus.

There is a lot of evidence that people in Britain have trouble with their colons. Cancer of the colon is the second most common cancer in the UK and as a nation we spend more than £50 million a year on laxatives to give our colons a boost. That indicates that a large majority of people in this country have sluggish colons that are not eliminating waste efficiently or safely.

Waste is passed through the colon and into the rectum by a series of muscular contractions, but if these contractions are a bit slow waste can start to build up. The refined carbohydrate, high fat diet that many of us eat also contributes to the problems of the toxic colon. If we eat such a diet for years on end, eat little in the way of fresh fruit and vegetables and include little fibre in our food, mucous and faecal matter become glued to the wall of a colon and pockets of debris accumulate.

If this happens, the bacterial flora of the colon will become unbalanced and allow hostile bacteria to flourish. The wall of the colon may be damaged, allowing harmful bacteria and viruses to invade the rest of the body. The group of viruses that are thought to cause ME, the enteroviruses, flourish in the intestine and they might have access to the rest of the body through a damaged colon wall.

Nutrients will not be absorbed through the wall of the colon that is coated with old faecal matter. Harmful toxins that would have been excreted may be absorbed back into the blood stream and taken to the liver for processing, therefore, the liver may be overwhelmed with toxins and other organs of the body may have to do the job of excreting them. For instance, the skin and the lungs may be used to do the job and this can result in bad breath, spots, unpleasant body odour and smelly feet.

These are just the short-term effects of a toxic colon. If the situation is allowed to carry on, this auto-intoxication can result in a wide variety of symptoms that has been described as like having a permanent hangover. In 1919 *The Lancet* published a paper describing the effects of auto-intoxication caused by a toxic colon. The paper by Sir W.A. Arbuthnot Lane, surgeon to the Royal Family, said that most of the ills of modern man stemmed from intestinal toxaemia. He wrote:

> The effect of auto-intoxication upon the brain and nervous system is very striking. Headache, varying in intensity, is a common symptom. I have known it so severe, and accompanied with such violent attacks of vomiting, as to lead a very distinguished neurologist to diagnose a cerebral tumour and to urge operative interference. Neuralgias are frequent and may involve a great variety of nerves. They may be very intense. Rheumatic pains are constantly complained of. The patient, while sleeping badly, may find it difficult to keep awake during the day. Bad dreams are frequent. On awakening in the morning the feeling experienced may be that of extreme prostration, no apparent benefit having been derived from the night's rest. The most distressing symptoms of auto-intoxication is the depression which so frequently accompanies it. It varies in severity from a feeling of mental incapacity to one which not infrequently leads the sufferer to terminate an existence which has become intolerable. All efforts at mental concentration are futile, while any physical exertion is followed by a period of complete exhaustion . . . The term 'neurasthenia' is very often applied to this condition of the nervous system . . . The patient loses control and fits of irritability or of violent passion are not infrequent. Such a person is difficult to live with. Many are supposed to be stupid, dull, inattentive, or even imbecile . . . The eyes are always affected. They afford an excellent and very delicate indication of the degree of auto-intoxication . . . They are due chiefly to degenerative processes in the lens and to loss of power in the ciliary muscle.

Some of those symptoms will be familiar to any ME sufferer: in fact that could be a text book description of ME.

At the time, Sir Arbuthnot Lane's description of auto-intoxication was met with much scepticism from the medical profession. He said: 'My explanation of the causation of a large number of diseases was regarded as being so simple and obvious as to be absurd.' The medical profession has ignored the concept of the toxic colon ever since. However, interest has been renewed in the past couple of years – more among alternative practitioners than among the conventional medical profession.

It is now possible to get help to deal with a toxic colon, but curing it takes time and patience. After many years of mistreating your colon you should not be surprised if it takes a few months to put things right. It needs a change in diet, the introduction of colon cleansing procedures and the use of herbs to keep the colon clean.

The quickest and easiest way to clean the colon is by using colon hydrotherapy or colonic irrigation. It is best to start off by going to a practitioner who is experienced in colonic irrigation – the Colonic International Association will help you to find one in your area. You will need a good sense of humour to go through with this as it is a technique that many people would find rather distasteful! A colonic therapist will insert a tube into your rectum through which water flows at a temperature to suit you. The water sluices around the colon dislodging any faecal material that is stuck to the wall of the colon. It is really a sophisticated enema except that old faeces can be removed while the water is pumped in. You would need just one cleansing session a week and should carry on until it is clear that no 'old' faeces are being removed – this would be at the stage where your new healthy diet and herbal cleansing remedies are beginning to take effect.

There is a do-it-yourself machine available but it is best to go to someone who is experienced in the technique before you try it yourself. Many people who have tried colonic therapy report that it gives them a light, healthy feeling inside.

In addition to colonic irrigation you should change the root cause of the problem: your diet. Many of the foods we eat today, particularly refined carbohydrates, dairy products and red meat, encourage stagnation of food in the digestive system leading to constipation. They also produce mucous when they are digested in the bowel which encourages them to stick to the colon wall. If food does not pass through the system quickly enough, or if it starts sticking to the walls of the intestine, it will accumulate in the colon and stay there sometimes for days at a time. Instead of being safely passed out of the body, toxins in the waste matter accumulate in the colon and eventually pass into the blood stream. The liver, which is the organ designed to deal with toxic wastes, becomes overwhelmed with these wastes from the colon that it would not normally have to deal with. If the liver is overwhelmed all sorts of symptoms might arise, similar to those described above.

One of the simplest ways of finding out if your colon is

accumulating toxic waste matter is to check your own body odour. If you have trouble with body odour, that is if you cannot keep smelling sweet with one bath a day, it is likely that you have a sluggish colon. If you have consistently bad breath that may also indicate a sluggish colon, although it is more likely to be a sign of tooth decay.

You might think the easy answer to all this is to swallow a few laxatives – but this is probably the worst thing you can do. Most laxatives work by irritating the bowel wall so that the muscular contractions increase the expulsion of food and the laxative as quickly as possible. Laxatives do nothing to loosen faecal matter from the bowel walls and, unfortunately, then tend to weaken the bowel muscles so that they only work when they are stimulated by yet another laxative.

Instead of using laxatives you should make changes to your diet to include as many fresh fruits and vegetables as possible. You should switch from white rice to brown, from white bread to wholemeal and try to include a wider variety of wholegrains in your diet. For instance, try rye bread instead of wheat bread. Try bulgur wheat instead of rice or try buckwheat or oat cakes instead of scones and toast, porridge and muesli instead of cornflakes and other refined cereals.

Some nutritionists believe you should avoid meat and dairy products if you are trying to keep your colon clean. Meat, eggs, milk, cheese, yogurt, butter, cream are all what are called mucoid-forming foods. They produce a lot of sticky mucous as they pass through the digestive tract that makes them stick more easily to the walls of the intestine. However, it would probably be wiser to add fruits, vegetables and wholegrain cereals to your diet rather than cut down too drastically on important sources of protein and energy. If you are eating a lot of fibrous foods these will help to keep your colon clean and free of waste build-up.

Some colonic practitioners and naturopaths will recommend herbal remedies that will help to clean the colon. The herbs may include chickweed, Irish moss, cloves, plantain, rosemary, bayberry bark and corn silk extract – or alternatives that have the same action. The basic mechanism is to regulate the bowel so that you have neither constipation nor diarrhoea. Herbs that dissolve mucous, purify the lymph system and the blood and soothe the stomach while all this is going on are also included. Some practitioners will advise the use of intestinal bulking agents that remove the material that has been loosened by the herbs.

135

One of the most common of these is psyllium husks which are now available in most good health stores. You should be sure to drink plenty of water on this programme as water is needed to help soften and carry away the hardened mucous and faeces.

There are some people who should not attempt colon cleansing. Pregnant women and anyone with inflammatory bowel disease, Crohn's disease or any other long-term bowel problem should avoid it.

As with any cleansing programme you may feel slightly unwell for the first couple of weeks. This is because toxins may be released from the faecal matter as it is dislodged from the walls of the intestine. Your faeces may have a foul odour for the first few weeks as old material is removed. Your abdomen may swell as old faeces swell with the water and bulking agents you might be taking. When the programme is complete your abdomen should be flatter than ever and you should be having regular bowel movements – at least once every day and sometimes twice.

Once you have been on a colon cleansing programme for a few weeks you should begin to notice the difference, if that was the root of your problem. You will feel clean. Your digestive system will be able to absorb more nutrients from your food as it is no longer blocked by mucous and stale faecal matter. It takes at least three to six months to cleanse the colon completely but this varies from person to person. At the same time, many practitioners would recommend you start regular skin brushing to stimulate the lymphoid system into removing toxins from the body. You can do this in the bath or shower with a loofa or long-handled brush and just scrub away until you feel invigorated.

15 Food and ME

Good nutrition is essential for recovery from ME. Many sufferers find they do not have much appetite and have little energy with which to prepare food. If this applies to you and it carries on for any length of time you could find yourself undernourished and incapable of making any attempt at recovery. You must make the effort to eat because without food your body cannot make the chemicals that fight infections and build up your immune system. If you really do not feel like eating, try with a small amount and then have another go later. If you do not eat you will feel worse later on and have even less of an appetite. If you carry on underfeeding yourself for any length of time your stomach will start to contract and then you might find it difficult to eat a whole meal. It is a vicious circle that you must try to avoid.

Protein

Foods with proteins are the most important ones in our diet. Every single cell in our body contains some kind of protein whether it is the protein of muscle, bone, cartilage, skin and blood. Every single enzyme in our body is made of a protein and many hormones are also proteins. They are used to make new body tissues, to replace worn-out tissues and to take the nutrients from one cell to another. The oxygen and nutrients in the blood are carried by proteins. A very important function of proteins is to make the antibodies that help us to fight disease causing bacteria and viruses – something that may be impaired in ME sufferers.

When you eat protein it is broken down into amino acids and rebuilt into the proteins that we use in the body. There are 22 amino acids and nine of them are essential. These are methionine, threonine, tryptophan, isoleucine, leucine, lysine, histadine, valine and phenylalanine. The other 13 amino acids can be made from these nine essential ones so it is not imperative that we eat foods that contain them in order to live.

Complete proteins are foods which contain all nine of the essential amino acids and they include animal proteins like meat, fish, poultry, dairy produce and eggs. But you do not have to eat these foods everyday to get an adequate supply of essential amino acids. Vegetables, beans and grains contain what are known as incomplete proteins. They contain small amounts of some, but not all, the essential amino acids. By combining different types of vegetable foods it is possible to get all the essential amino acids. What one food lacks in one type of amino acid another will supply, for instance, in Japan a meal of rice and tofu (made from soya bean curd) will supply all essential amino acids without eating meat products. In Mexico, beans and rice is a national dish and also a meal that provides complete proteins. So it is not necessary to eat meat or animal products to obtain all the protein you need as long as you combine foods that between them contain complete protein.

You do need to eat protein every day. There is nowhere in the body to store protein and after just one day without it your body will start to break down the protein in non-essential tissues like muscles and use it to supply protein to organs like the liver, the brain and kidneys that are essential for survival. In ME sufferers who have muscle fatigue it may be particularly important to eat protein. If protein in the muscles is being broken down it will weaken them still further and slow down recovery.

The best way to supply your body with protein is throughout the day in small regular meals. If you give your body all its daily protein in one go, some will go to waste as the body copes better with smaller amounts eaten more frequently. Four or five small meals a day would be better than a single massive intake at one main meal.

The amount of protein you need depends on your age, weight, sex and state of health. Even if you are eating an adequate amount of protein, being ill, or under stress or very inactive can make you lose more protein than you synthesise for use in the body. If you are very inactive your muscles start to waste away. Not only is your body losing water and fat but vital proteins as well and if you lose excessive amounts of protein this can result in severe side effects like fever, pain and diarrhoea.

If you are ill your ability to absorb proteins may also be impaired, so you may find it advisable to take free-form amino acids. These can be extremely helpful for ME patients who have trouble digesting protein because for all intents and purposes they are pre-digested. They pass quickly and easily through the gut wall into the bloodstream.

Carbohydrates

Many people think of carbohydrates as little more than basic

138

foods that fill you up. But there is more to it than that. Carbohydrates are a very important part of the diet and you would soon fall ill if you stopped eating them altogether.

There are two types of carbohydrate: the starches, which are the complex carbohydrates found in cereals, grains and beans; and the sugars, or simple carbohydrates found in fruits and vegetables.

Another distinction is between natural and refined carbohydrates. Natural carbohydrates are foods as they are found in nature, without anything taken away, for instance potatoes with their skins on or wholemeal flours. Refined carbohydrates are extracted from their natural sources and either eaten on their own or added to other foods. White sugar, white flour, some breakfast cereals and instant potato mix are all examples of refined carbohydrates.

All ME sufferers should ensure that they eat complex, unrefined carbohydrates in preference to refined ones. While all carbohydrates provide the body with energy, in the form of glucose, if that energy is provided in its simple form for instance as white sugar, the body uses this energy up very quickly leading to feelings of fatigue, lethargy, headaches, and extreme hunger or nausea. But if the glucose is provided in the form of complex carbohydrate, for instance wholemeal bread or baked potatoes, that has to be digested before it can be used, you will get a slow, steady release of energy rather than huge ups and downs.

Many ME sufferers seem to have problems with hypoglycaemia (which we have discussed in Chapter 6) and almost all report fluctuations in mood, some on a practically hourly basis. If they were to cut down on their sugar intake and remove coffee and tea from their diet they would be in much better shape.

The best way to avoid soaring and plummeting blood sugar levels which will play havoc with your system and your emotions is to avoid refined carbohydrates and eat several small meals of protein and complex carbohydrate throughout the day. That will keep your blood sugar virtually constant and avoid the possibility that it will drop to very low levels.

Hypoglycaemia is caused by over-production of insulin, the hormone that controls the metabolism of sugar and other carbohydrates. When we eat concentrated amounts of sugar the levels of blood sugar rise and the pancreas produces insulin. The insulin clears the blood of this excess sugar by taking it to the cells of the body where it is used for energy or is converted into fat for storage.

The body was not designed to deal with very high concentrations of sugar. When we eat sugar the body gears up for more food to follow close behind so it releases enough insulin to handle a whole meal. That often turns out to be more than enough and so too much sugar is cleared from the blood leading to weakness, faintness, shakiness, confusion, irritability and extreme hunger. That is why if you snack on bars of chocolate you will feel a rush of energy as soon as the sugar is absorbed, followed a couple of hours later by the symptoms of hypoglycaemia.

This reactive hypoglycaemia will happen to most people who eat sugary foods between meals or who have very long gaps between meals. Eating a lot of refined carbohydrate is the most common cause of this condition. Chronic stress, food allergies, an under- or over-active thyroid gland, deficiencies of the minerals zinc, magnesium, potassium, manganese, some medicines, missed meals, cigarette smoking and excessive tea and coffee consumption may all contribute to it.

Angela, for instance, whose case history we recounted at the beginning of this book, used to eat lots of sweet foods. 'I had cravings for chocolate,' she says, 'quite strong cravings in fact. Halfway through the morning I would want to go out and buy a Mars Bar because I felt I didn't have enough energy to carry on through the morning. I also used to drink lots of coffee – in fact I sometimes had as many as six cups in a morning. Almost as soon as I had finished one I felt as if I needed another.'

Another problem with eating refined carbohydrates is that most of the nutrients will have been removed during processing. For instance, an ordinary potato with its skin contains carbohydrates, protein, iron, the vitamins thiamine, niacin, vitamin C and vitamin B6, as well as the minerals phosphorus, copper, magnesium and iodine – all vital for health. By the time a potato has had its skin removed, been doused in fat and cooked at high temperatures to make a packet of crips, much of those nutrients will have been lost and a great deal of extra calories will have been added in the form of fat.

The phrase 'empty calories' is associated with refined carbohydrates because by the time many of us come to eat these foods they have very little nutritional value left. A good example of a healthy food that is virtually destroyed by processing is wheat bread. Up to 80 per cent of the original nutrients are removed from the wheat to make white flour and while legislation in the UK requires bakers to add some vitamins to white flour to restore some of the nutrients, white bread and white flour products are not a whole food.

Natural carbohydrates are also good sources of dietary fibre, which provides the roughage that keeps the digestive system running smoothly and helps us to get rid of waste products more efficiently. Refined carbohydrates generally have all the fibre removed so they no longer perform this vital function.

Carbohydrates provide the body's main energy source: glucose. Glucose is the main fuel source for muscles and it is what the brain needs to work properly. If you do not eat enough carbohydrates your body is forced to burn fats and protein for its energy, a potentially dangerous situation. Without carbohydrates, fats burn very inefficiently, producing poisonous waste products called ketones. These ketones accumulate in the blood and can produce a variety of effects including nausea, fatigue and apathy and they can even, in severe cases, damage the brain. Your kidneys are also put under more pressure as they have the job of removing these ketones before they do too much damage.

There is a wide range of whole grains and cereals on the market now and it is well worth trying some of them out. Bulgur wheat, millet, barley, brown rice, buckwheat, wholemeal pasta are all whole cereals that you can now find in the supermarket. Many dried beans and peas are valuable sources of carbohydrate as well as protein.

Although ME sufferers would be wise to eat plenty of carbohydrates that does not mean plenty of sugar. The only value sugar has is to provide you with calories, which is all right as long as you are going to use all those calories. The main problem for ME sufferers is that refined and even unrefined sugars contain so few nutrients as to be almost valueless. As an ME sufferer it is essential that you eat those foods that give you nutrients.

Fats

Most of us eat far too much fat and ME sufferers are unlikely to be any exception. Our daily requirement for dietary fat is about one tablespoon of polyunsaturated fat. But many of us eat about eight times that amount of fat in one day and most of that is the kind we should be avoiding: saturated fat. One of the reasons for this is that many of the foods we eat for protein, for instance beef, pork and lamb, have a very high fat content and so we probably eat more than we realise. Fats are a very concentrated source of energy for the body but pound for pound they contain many more calories than an equivalent weight of proteins and carbohydrates.

On the plus side, fats do sometimes help to make food more appetising and, as they take longer to digest, they help to stop you feeling hungry so quickly after a meal.

Although we almost all eat too much fat we could not do without it entirely as it plays an important role in some of the body mechanisms. Body fat helps to cushion the internal organs and protects them from injury. It also helps insulate against changes in temperature as it is a poor conductor of heat. Which is why thin people feel the cold faster than fat ones and why Channel swimmers are almost all rotund.

But the only fats you really need to eat are polyunsaturated ones. In particular, they are a source of the essential fatty acid, linoleic acid, which the body uses to make other fats. It is in order to provide extra essential fatty acids (or EFAs as they are known) that some ME sufferers take evening primrose oil. This is an oil which is extracted from the seeds of the evening primrose, a plant that can be grown widely in Britain, and a product which Dr Jenkins and a small number of other practitioners and nutritionists prescribe for patients with ME. It is thought to be particularly effective for patients with multiple sclerosis because it is suspected that they often have a deficiency of EFAs and, in particular, of gammalinolenic acid. It is this which is converted in the body to the important prostaglandin PGE1. Evening primrose oil is unique in that it is the only plant source to contain gammalinolenic acid.

In her book, *Evening Primrose Oil*, Judy Graham, who suffers from MS herself, describes some of the oil's properties:

1. It stimulates the T-lymphocytes, the white cells which are the most important part of the body's immune system.
2. It stops the platelets clumping together.
3. It makes faulty red blood cells return to normal. (Both this and its effects on the platelets is interesting because researchers in Australia have discovered that a high percentage of people with ME have red blood cell abnormalities. *Time*, in its Australian edition in September 1987, disclosed that deformed red blood cells had been found in 90 per cent of the ME patients who had been studied.)

4. It produces increased mobility, increased walking ability, improved eyesight, relief of constipation and reduced spasm (all of which are symptoms that certainly occur in people with MS and, to some degree, occur also in people with ME).

This slight similarity with multiple sclerosis is an interesting one and it may be that the other similarities will be noticed when a joint endeavour of the ME Action Campaign and ARMS, the MS charity, gets under way. The plan, at the time of writing, is for the ME Action Campaign to share space in not less than 58 therapy centres around the country which at the moment are run exclusively by ARMS.

The problem with evening primrose oil, unless you are fortunate enough to find a rare doctor who can prescribe it on the National Health, is that it is expensive. Six to eight capsules a day are needed, divided into three separate doses, and they should be taken over a period of months. (They should be stopped, however, for two weeks on either side of an EPD injection if the sufferer is receiving that particular treatment). At the time of writing it has just been announced that from now on evening primrose oil may be prescribed on the National Health for patients with eczema. It remains to be seen whether it will ever be extended to those with ME.

Vitamins and Minerals
In an ideal world, if you were eating a healthy, well-balanced diet there would be no need to take extra vitamins and minerals. But it is likely that because you are not in full health you will need more of them than the normal person. Sometimes people who are ill cannot absorb or metabolise nutrients as efficiently as those in full health so people with ME would be wise to make sure they eat a highly nutritious diet and take supplements in addition.

Vitamins: essential for good health because they are involved in many of the body's chemical reactions. They help to process other nutrients like proteins and carbohydrates, they help to form blood cells, hormones, genetic material found in every cell of the body, and chemicals that are important in the nervous system. They also help enzymes carry out their various roles in the body. There are 13 vitamins that are officially recognised as essential to good health and they are split into two groups: fat soluble and water soluble.

Vitamins A, D, E and K: these are called the fat soluble vitamins and are stored in the body fat. There is no need to eat them every day as long as you get enough each week to keep the stored levels topped up. In fact, if you eat too many, they can build up to toxic levels so you should be wary of taking excessive supplements of fat soluble vitamins.

Vitamin A: is important in maintaining healthy eyes, skin, hair, bone growth and teeth development. Some researchers have linked a vitamin A deficiency in countries where there is a low intake of green and yellow vegetables with a high incidence of cancers of the mouth, stomach and colon. Vitamin A is found in many foods: major sources are animal produce, particularly liver, kidney, eggs, milk and butter, where it is found as the complete form of the vitamin. In addition, green, yellow, red and orange fruits and vegetables are good sources of beta carotene which is made into vitamin A in the body. Generally, the darker the colour of the vegetable or fruit the higher the beta carotene content. Good sources are carrots, spinach, cabbage, red peppers and oranges.

Vitamin D: is essential for the absorption of calcium and phosphorus which are important in bone formation and maintenance. It increases our absorption of these two minerals from the food we eat and helps to lay them down in the bone. In the kidneys vitamin D helps to reabsorb calcium and phosphate from the urine so that we do not lose too much. There are many foods that contain it, including milk, eggs, fatty fishes like tuna and mackerel, cod liver oil, butter, cheese and margarines (in the UK vitamins A and D must be added to margarine by law). But most of our vitamin D intake comes from exposure to sunlight, which activates chemicals in the skin to produce it. Because of this most of us do not need supplemental vitamin D in the summer or autumn. But in the winter and spring, when our resources are depleted by the dark days of January and February, additional vitamin D is a good idea.

Vitamin E: helps to form red blood cells and muscle cells and one of its most important roles is as an anti-oxidant. Our cells are very sensitive to the damaging effects of oxygen and things called free radicals that break down the cell constituents by oxidising them. Vitamin E helps to stop this. Most vegetable oils, wholewheat and other wholegrain cereals, dried beans and green leafy vegetables contain vitamin E.

Vitamin K: helps to produce blood clotting factors and assists in normal bone metabolism. Green leafy vegetables, peas, potatoes and liver provide some of our daily needs. But an important source of vitamin K is produced by the bacteria that live in the small bowel of our digestive system. If you suffer from Candida overgrowth and you do not eat enough vitamin-K-rich foods you may be at risk of a deficiency as the normal gut flora is disturbed.

The water-soluble vitamins are C (ascorbic acid) and the eight B vitamins – B1 (thiamine), B2 (riboflavin), B3 (niacin or nicotinic acid), B5 (pantothenic acid), B6 (pyridoxine), B12 (cobalamine), and folic acid and biotin.
   The water-soluble vitamins are different from the fat-soluble in that they do not need fat to be absorbed into the body and they are not generally stored in the body. As they are all soluble in water these vitamins are lost through the urine and sweat and for this reason you need to make sure you take in B and C vitamins every day.

Vitamin B1: (thiamine) is crucial to the function of heart and skeletal muscle and plays an important role in the brain, kidney and liver. All these organs and tissues have high energy requirements and vitamin B1 helps to release energy from carbohydrates. Some of the chemicals used by the nerves are also produced with its help. B1 deficiency soon leads to mental confusion, muscular weakness and swelling of the heart, and considering the importance of muscle function in ME all sufferers should make sure they have an adequate intake. It is widely distributed in many vegetable and animal foods; good sources are whole grains, pork, beef, oysters, lentils, brown rice and other whole grains. Refined grains and cereals have considerably reduced amounts.

Vitamin B2: (riboflavin) helps to release energy from carbohydrates, proteins and fats and increases the metabolism of vitamin B6. It also helps to form some important enzymes in the liver which are involved in our metabolism. Milk and dairy produce, meats, especially liver, dark green vegetables, dried peas and beans are all good sources.

Vitamin B3: (niacin or nicotinic acid and nicotinamide) produces energy in the cells along with vitamins B1 and B2 by assisting in the production of key enzymes. Meat, especially beef, fish, milk, eggs and wholegrain cereals are important sources. B3 can also be synthesised from the amino acid tryptophan.

Vitamin B5: (pantothenic acid) helps to form hormones and nerve regulating chemicals as well as assisting the other B vitamins in energy production from carbohydrates, proteins and fats. It is widely distributed in foods but particularly high levels are found in liver and other meats, eggs and wholegrain cereals. Pantothenic acid, or calcium pantothenate as it is sometimes called, is very important for people who are under stress, which means it is particularly helpful to sufferers of ME.

Vitamin B6: (pyridoxine) plays a major role in the metabolism of protein and amino acids and the two are very closely related. The more protein you eat the more vitamin B6 you need to metabolise it. B6 helps produce some important chemicals in the body and is important in normal brain chemistry; a deficiency of B6 often shows itself in changes in mood such as depression. It helps our body to absorb some essential minerals, particularly zinc and magnesium, and it also regulates the metabolism of essential fatty acids. Wholegrain cereals, meat, fish, eggs, avocados, bananas, nuts, potatoes and green leafy vegetables are important food sources.

Vitamin B12: is one of the few water-soluble vitamins that is stored in the body and is vital for the production of red blood cells, which is why failure to absorb it is a major cause of pernicious anaemia. Good sources are offal, meat, some fish, dairy produce, eggs and brewer's yeast. B12 is not found in any vegetables so strict vegetarians – vegans who do not eat any animal produce – risk a deficiency.

Folic acid: is found frequently in green leafy vegetables and indeed that is where it gets its name from – foliage. It is closely linked with B12 and is important in the nervous system. It is also stored in the liver but the body's store has only three to six months' supply. Many of the foods that contain vitamin B12 also contain folic acid, for instance liver and offal, and it is also very common in green leafy vegetables. It has been discovered that many psychiatric patients have deficiencies of folic acid and the B vitamins in general. Anyone who suffers depression should be sure to eat enough of these vitamins.

Biotin: is thought to contribute to the formation of essential fatty acids in the body but not very much is known about this vitamin.

It is widely distributed in meats, egg yolk, dairy produce and dark green vegetables.

Vitamin C: has very many roles in the body. It helps form collagen that is the basis for connective tissue and bones. It is essential for cholesterol metabolism and helps produce cortisol from the adrenal gland and the hormone noradrenalin. It is thought to prevent the production of chemicals that may cause cancer although that is not fully established. It may also be involved in helping the body to fight off viral infections. Some doctors have used high doses of vitamin C to treat viral hepatitis, polio, measles, mumps, viral pneumonia, meningitis, and shingles. There have been few clinical trials to assess the efficacy of vitamin C in curing these diseases but the anecdotal evidence is impressive.

Everyone has different needs for vitamin C. It is likely that ME sufferers will have an increased need for it as it is well recognised that people who are under stress or suffering from infection need more vitamin C. Most fruits and green vegetables (including broccoli, brussels sprouts and cauliflower) contain it. Liver, kidney and potatoes are also good sources. Rosehips, black-currants, blackberries and citrus fruits have very high levels.

Reading through these descriptions you will notice that several foods crop up time and time again as good sources of vitamins. Liver, green vegetables and wholegrain cereals are some of the most important sources of these essential nutrients. Many people have an aversion to liver because it does not look very nice but it is such a valuable source of vitamins that it would be worthwhile for any ME sufferer to get to like this food. You do not have to eat it every day, but a portion of liver once a week would provide you, for instance, with much of the vitamin A you need all in one go. By including plenty of wholegrain cereals, fresh fruit and green vegetables in your diet you will go a long way to avoiding sub-optimum levels of vitamins.

However, it is important to remember that vitamins can be lost from food by bad storage and cooking. There are several things you can do to make sure you get the maximum benefit from your food. Buy fresh or frozen fruit and vegetables rather than canned produce which may have up to half the vitamins leached out during cooking and canning in fluid. Shop often for fresh produce and try not to store things for too long before eating them. Avoid soaking fresh vegetables before cooking, boil them in the minimum amount of water needed and cook until just tender to avoid vitamins leaching into the water. Keep the water for gravy. Cook potatoes in their skins. Do not cut vegetables too small – it is estimated that cutting a potato in half leaves just 31 per cent of the original vitamin C content. Pressure cooking or using a microwave oven to cook vegetables significantly cuts down on the loss of vitamins because of the short cooking time.

Minerals
Minerals are inorganic substances that play a vital role in many of the body's functions such as acting as catalysts in enzyme reactions. The macrominerals include calcium, phosphorus, magnesium and chlorine and are the bulk elements that are needed in large quantities (several hundred milligrams a day). The trace elements include iron, zinc, copper, manganese, iodine, chromium, selenium, molybdenum, cobalt and sulphur. They are needed in minute quantities. Some, like copper, are potent poisons if they are present in large quantities.

The relationship between minerals and other nutrients is very complex. Some minerals enhance the uptake of others; if there is too little magnesium in the diet, the absorption of calcium, for instance, is impaired. An excess of some minerals may decrease the absorption of others; an example of this is zinc which will prevent the uptake of copper if it is present in too large quantities and can actually cause a copper deficiency. Sometimes too few vitamins will prevent you absorbing all the minerals you need from your food; an inadequate vitamin C intake, for example, will inhibit the absorption of a number of minerals, especially iron.

It is beyond the scope of this book to analyse each mineral in detail, although their importance in health is under-recognised in this country. Pregnant women, for instance, are routinely given iron supplements, but too much iron can inhibit the absorption of zinc which is an important mineral during pregnancy. Very few doctors have the facilities to measure their patients' mineral status but some private practitioners and nutritionists will analyse sweat and blood samples and then recommend dietary changes, or a course of supplements, that will correct mineral imbalances. Sweat sampling is thought to be one of the best ways of measuring the levels of some minerals, such as zinc, in the body and blood samples are used for others. It is now believed that samples of hair will not give quite such a useful measurement of your mineral status so it would be better to consult a practitioner who does not base his whole analysis on hair sampling.

In our description of important minerals we have limited the discussion to minerals that may be most important in ME and those in which sufferers are most likely to be deficient. Some minerals, such as phosphorus, are so abundant in our diets that deficiency is rarely likely to be a problem.

Calcium: this is sometimes thought to be important in the context of ME sufferers who also have food allergies. People who are on an elimination diet for the management of their allergies are thought by some to risk calcium deficiency if they are told to cut out dairy produce. But there are plenty of other foods rich in calcium including broccoli, legumes, green leafy vegetables, nuts, sesame seeds, peas, beans and lentils and if you eat plenty of these you will get adequate calcium even if you are not eating milk, butter or cheese.

A big problem with ME is that you may be taking very little exercise. If you are immobile, particularly if you are confined to bed, calcium will be lost from your bones. Some sort of exercise in the form of yoga, which sufferers do not find so exhausting, may be useful in maintaining your calcium status. If you are taking calcium supplements it is important to choose ones that will be readily absorbed by the body. Calcium lactate, gluconate or sulphate or amino-chelated calcium are some of the best forms to take.

Magnesium: closely linked with calcium and phosphorus in the body, a deficiency can cause a wide range of problems including weakness and tiredness, hypoglycaemia, nausea, muscle cramps, insomnia, confusion and disorientation, constipation, numbness and tingling and a range of psychiatric symptoms. When you go to your practitioner with ME you may be tested for magnesium deficiency as some of the symptoms are similar to those of ME and it seems that almost all ME sufferers – and indeed most allergy patients – are deficient in both zinc and magnesium. It may be that they are unable to retain within their bodies a normal proportion of the zinc or magnesium from their diet. Rich sources of magnesium include green leafy vegetables, whole grains, nuts, shrimps and soya beans.

Iron: important for ME sufferers because one of the symptoms of a deficiency is muscle fatigue and tiredness. If you are short of iron your muscles will be further hampered, so you need to sort this out to give your muscles the best possible chance to recover. Iron deficiency is the commonest mineral deficiency but it is underestimated and under-recognised. Studies among English women aged 15 to 25 have revealed they were getting only 70 to 75 per cent of the recommended daily intake. Such a chronic deficiency gives rise to chronic fatigue, listlessness, a very rapid heartbeat on exertion (more than you would expect), concave nails and difficulty with swallowing. Often these symptoms resolve themselves within a few days of taking iron supplements. Rich sources are offal, egg yolk, legumes, shell fish, parsley, cocoa and molasses. Refined carbohydrates and milk are poor sources of iron while meat, fish and poultry and green vegetables have medium amounts.

Zinc: this is fast becoming recognised as one of the most important minerals in our diet and many conditions have been attributed to zinc deficiency. It is involved in the smooth running of more than 100 enzyme reactions. Signs of a severe deficiency are behavioural and sleep disturbances, immune deficiencies, white spots on fingernails, impaired taste or smell, hair loss and diarrhoea.

Zinc plays an important role in immune function and this is one reason why every ME sufferer should either make sure their diet contains enough or should supplement it. If you do not get enough zinc the thymus gland stops functioning properly and it is the thymus that produces the lymphocytes, the cells involved in fighting infections. Animals and people with a zinc deficiency have an increased susceptibility to infections because they have fewer lymphocytes.

Zinc deficiency is also thought to play a part in the depression of the immune system seen after a bereavement or other very stressful life events such as giving birth and anyone who has a depressed immune system, as ME sufferers do, would benefit from zinc supplementation. An easy way of telling if you have deficiency is to buy a solution of zinc and put a few drops in a very small amount of water. If you can taste the solution you probably have enough zinc. If you cannot taste it you should take zinc supplements for a while and test yourself once a week until you can taste a solution. After that you should test yourself at regular intervals to make sure you do not fall short. If you take a zinc supplement you should try and take it at least one hour before or after mealtimes, in order for it to be absorbed most efficiently.

Fresh oysters are the best source of dietary zinc. Lamb chops, steak, fresh liver, split peas, egg yolk, whole grain cereals, garlic, carrots, beans, and nuts are all very good sources.

Easy Eating
It is all very well having a thorough knowledge of nutrition but many people with ME say they do not have the physical energy to cook and eat a meal. This is where you have to use all your resources to think of ways of making it easy. If you have a family they may have to take more of the burden of cooking, with you perhaps just giving instructions. Do not feel guilty about this; just explain clearly what you can and cannot do and explain how your energy varies from day-to-day.

If you feel you cannot face the effort of preparing a whole meal then don't. Do a bit now, rest, then do a bit more later. Or choose foods that do not need preparing. For instance, a meal of baked potatoes, grilled chicken and salad needs little more than popping in the oven and washing a few vegetables. Don't peel foods that don't really need it. Potatoes taste better in their skins and are more nutritious. Cook two batches of rice in one go and freeze one portion for another time. All you have to do is thaw it out, pour boiling water over it to heat, and strain it. Many ME sufferers complain that they do not have the energy to peel potatoes or make a salad, when what they are really saying is that they feel weak and tired if they *stand* while peeling potatoes and making salads. The answer is to *sit* and if you do not have a kitchen stool then do it at the dining table or even when sitting in an easy chair in the living-room.

There are plenty of things you can do to cut down the work in the kitchen – all it needs is a little thought. Best of all would be to read Leslie Kenton's book *Raw Energy* and realise just how delicious food can be raw. It is much more nutritious and, of course, it means a lot less expenditure of energy.

Almost all ME patients who have made a considerable recovery are people who have paid a great deal of attention to their diet and to good nutrition. Those who defiantly stick to habits accumulated over a lifetime because they claim it is too late to change will seldom make any progress.

16   Grounds for Optimism

Most doctors and patients would agree there is no recognised cure for ME. But some people do make a considerable recovery and the remarkable thing about the people who get better is that, for the most part, they have used completely different approaches. There is no one remedy that anyone could point to and say, 'Yes, that is what cured me.'

Some have benefited from allergy testing, others have successfully used the anti-Candida approach. Some have rushed from doctor to doctor in the search for the right drug only to find that what they really needed was complete rest. Some sufferers have found anti-depressants useful and homoeopathy has helped others. But for all, adopting a positive attitude has been the key to dealing with their illness. For most people the key to recovery from ME is coming to terms with it and finding curative methods that suit them, The case histories that follow have been included to demonstrate that it is possible to make a substantial recovery from ME.

Case History 1
In 1984, 22-year-old Nicky Spurgeon was Britain's Number 4 women's squash player. She was 5' 9" tall, athletic and strong, and had a reputation for fitness in a game which puts an emphasis on supreme fitness. She ran 10 miles a day, played at least one competitive game of squash every day, and then spent a further 2–3 hours training. 'I was known as one of the fittest women in the sport,' she says.

Three months later Nicky couldn't play at all.

At Christmas time that year I came down with 'flu and just couldn't seem to shake it off. I had just won my first major tournament and was feeling a lot of pressure from the press to win again three weeks later. I lost and felt depressed about it and, looking back at that time of my life now, I realised I was probably over-training – as some athletes do.

152

After going down with the 'flu virus I just never seemed to be able to recover my strength. My symptoms went from bad to worse. If I tried to play squash, I could not do very much and then immediately afterwards I would feel 'out of it', incredibly tired. The next day I would feel even worse. I found that I could play for a bit but that if I pushed myself too far the symptoms would come on really suddenly, my legs would turn to jelly and I just couldn't do any more. It was not a question of giving up or not *wanting* to play any more, I just *couldn't*. It would suddenly become physically impossible to continue.

I had to sleep 12–14 hours a day, suffered from muscle ache in the upper back and neck, had ringing in the ears, bad dreams, cold feet and hands and, on a bad day, would lose my co-ordination and become very clumsy. I would hit the kerb while driving, walk into the side of doors and just generally seem to be incapable of doing things quite right.

It got so bad that I was unable to take any exercise at all – even walking up a flight of stairs was exhausting. When I began to get a little better, I found I could exercise a tiny amount but as soon as I did enough to make my muscles ache I felt extremely unwell and this seemed to bring back all my symptoms. At first I was falling asleep all over the place, practically every hour. It felt very much like the fatigue I had with glandular fever when I was young. Too much cooking or even a walk could reduce me to tears with fatigue and hurting muscles. I felt irritable, I found difficulty finding the correct words when speaking, and suffered from terrible hunger if I ever missed a meal.

I saw a doctor who put me on a diet of only chicken and rice and after being on it for three weeks or so I realised that I had become allergic to the rice and it was making me ill. I saw other doctors and had many tests, including one at St Mary's Hospital, Paddington to look for evidence of a Coxsackie-B virus. It was negative. I also had exhaustive tests at a Sports Clinic in Germany run by two very sympathetic doctors who knew me from my squash activities. They could only say that, although they believed there was definitely something wrong, they could not find out what it was. What they did establish was that during exercise I was producing too much lactic acid in my muscles.

Things got worse and worse and I felt that *no one* was helping me. I felt that everyone, even my doctor and family, were sitting back and watching me sink deeper and deeper into depression. I had no idea what to do or how to help myself. I was so angry and frustrated and in such despair that I punched my fist through a plate-glass window.

After that I was bundled off to see a psychiatrist, who by coincidence happened to have been an assistant to Dr Melvin Ramsay at the time of the ME outbreak at the Royal Free Hospital. She suggested I tried an anti-depressant called dothiepin (brand name Prothiaden). It's a tricyclic anti-depressant and comes in 25 mg capsules. For some time it seemed to make little difference and so the doctor suggested I increase the dosage. It took me a long time to get the dosage right, but eventually we settled on what is reckoned to be a high amount: 150 mg to be taken all in one go at bedtime. I have been on it two years now and I must say that it does seem to have helped. Twice in that period I have left the bottle of capsules behind when travelling and each time without it I quickly went back to how I was before: feeling completely out of it, confused, woozy and extremely fatigued.

Nicky's story is a remarkable one in that she seems to have found two things that helped. One was dothiepin and the other was something that came completely out of the blue. On a visit to Barbados she met and fell in love with the famous West Indian cricketer Sir Garfield Sobers. She now spends most of her time in Barbados and says that the warm, sunny climate has definitely helped her. So, of course, must have her relationship, especially as she was with somebody to whom exercise was a way of life. Slowly, she began to be able to exercise again, first of all by playing a few holes of golf and then gradually increasing the amount of exercise very carefully. Less than a year ago she found it was still out of the question to exercise every day. But now she is coaching squash players and even going for 2–3 mile runs. If she exercises two days in succession she still feels extremely tired on the third day and finds that every time she takes exercise she must nap for at least 20 minutes to a half-hour immediately afterwards. Nicky has other comments to make about her health which will sound strange to most healthy people but will be familiar to people suffering from ME.

'There seems to be a strange pattern. I will feel very bad and very low a day before feeling better. And vice-versa: I will feel great and think I am back to my old self the day before feeling lousy. I also have to be careful not to undersleep and not to oversleep as either can leave me feeling awful.'

Case History 2

A 39-year-old male, a director in a vegetable growing business, has suffered from ME for four years. He reports his major symptoms as having extreme breathing difficulties and fatigue. 'Some mornings,' he says 'I feel so tired it is as though I have never been to sleep.'

The onset of his symptoms was quite sudden. In October 1984 he went swimming and noticed the water felt very cold and that, try as he could, however frantically he swam, he just could not seem to get warm. Then a cough started which would not go away, and just before Christmas he got what seemed like a severe attack of 'flu: aching limbs, dizziness, a fever and increasing feebleness.

Naturally I thought I was starting the 'flu but by Christmas it was obvious that whatever I had, it most certainly was not 'flu. I was dizzy, feeble beyond belief, aching all over, but worst of all I could not breathe, other than at a very shallow level. I was getting long coughing fits that produced no phlegm and reduced me to a wreck. I am told that my face went grey and stayed that colour for the next 12 months. I was unable to do any work that involved even minor exertion. If I exerted myself at all I felt as though a vice had been tightened on my windpipe.

The 'flu symptoms gradually faded, but shivering bouts which lasted 24 hours would occur every two or three weeks.

I lost a half-stone in weight, even though normally I am just over nine stone. I had ringing in my ears for six months and I began to think I needed my eyes tested as I had headaches behind my eyes. Bright light bothered me and I had to start wearing sun glasses.

I have always been strong, a swift walker and a few years ago I completed a 50-mile walk in one day. Even though I had lost the kind of fitness necessary for that I could still walk long distances easily, but after Christmas 1984 a walk, or should I say a stroll, of only 100 yards or so would leave me sitting on a wall or tree stump gasping for air, a total wreck.

The physical symptoms that lasted longest were the breathing problems, the feebleness and the awful, grinding fatigue. Even now I can fall asleep anywhere, something that never happened before all this started. I had always been very active so the enforced inactivity was a terrible shock to me. I lost all drive and ambition, just doing as much as I had to do to keep things ticking over. It was as though I was cruising in a state of semi-consciousness. Somehow, I am not sure how, I have got a little better and now, nearly three years later, I feel I am just beginning to come alive again.

Case History 3

Hilary McLennan became ill in April 1986 during her second year at London University. Her major cerebral symptoms were lack of concentration, loss of memory and slow movements. Physically, she had muscular fatigue and extreme exhaustion. She was, she says, 'absolutely exhausted. I couldn't do anything. I wasn't hungry, I couldn't eat anything. I lost about two-and-a-half stone. I was unable to think at all. Even simple little tasks were beyond me. My mind was an absolute blank and I just lay in bed like a vegetable. I was sleeping 19 hours a day.'

Hilary went to one of the university doctors but got little sympathy. When she told the doctor she was so thirsty that she was drinking as much as one-and-a-half litres every 20 minutes the doctor merely told her: 'Well, the weather is pretty hot at the moment isn't it? That probably explains it.' The weather was also blamed for her needing to sleep 19 hours a day and the doctor concluded by telling her to 'adopt a positive attitude and get on with life.'

Three days later she collapsed and went to her parents' home in Surrey. There she was lucky. Hilary was one of the few ME sufferers fortunate enough to have had the same GP for many years and, since the GP had known Hilary since she was a child, she knew she was not a shirker who wanted to escape from life. She knew and trusted Hilary enough to realise her symptoms were genuine. If she said she was totally, utterly and completely exhausted, then she was. She was not someone who would put it all on.

Hilary's GP knew a little about ME and what she didn't know she found out from Professor Mowbray in London and Dr Behan in Glasgow. On the basis of her unusual symptoms Hilary was diagnosed as having ME. Her doctor did not prescribe any pills, she did not look for a miracle cure. What she did do was take the trouble to talk the subject through with both Hilary and her mother (who has a PhD in Botany). The result was a practical, dispassionate, almost scientific look at what the illness was.

We're a very unsentimental family (says Hilary, who has two brothers and a sister). There were no tears and no fuss was made. There was little emotion involved, it was all discussed very practically – which helped, for instance, when it came to the question of using a wheelchair. I'd been in bed most of the time and was feeling a bit better and wanted to get about and into the world a bit more. A wheelchair seemed the ideal answer. There were no psychological connotations. I didn't spend a lot of time thinking about how people would react to me or whether I would feel like a cripple or anything like that. We just decided it would be the best way to get around.

Even so, Hilary says recovery was a very slow process. Her mother played a very important role and, she says, 'channelled my emotions in a positive direction. She's a very positive person and there was no doubt in her mind that I would recover.'

Nearly two years after she first contracted ME, Hilary heard that the BBC was planning a *Horizon* programme on the subject. She wrote them a letter saying there was a need for positive comment and how important it was to put across the message that you could take steps to help yourself in the light of the apathy shown by doctors.

It must have impressed *Horizon* because they went down to film her shortly afterwards. A few months later Hilary had improved a lot and says:

Even at the time of the Horizon piece I felt I was just staggering around in the spaghetti of my brain. When I was really bad it seemed as if the virus had got into my brain tissue so badly that I couldn't spin words together and the wrong ones would come out. Now one of the best things is that I can read properly again. I still can't write for very long because after a bit my forearms ache so much. I can do things that don't take too long but I still can't do anything that takes sustained effort. Even so, I'm going back to university next year to finish my degree course in anthropology.

Case History 4

Romily Gregory was a 29-year-old charity worker helping refugees to find homes in Britain when, in May 1985, she had a mild bout of 'flu that turned into ME.

It was the weekend before I was due to go on a week's holiday to Ibiza with a friend. I got a mild bout of 'flu but decided to go all the same. Although I was feeling a bit funny and I had to sleep quite a lot I did things like windsurfing and I was still well enough to hire mopeds and bomb around Ibiza. Then I got back and I remember thinking 'Oh, I'll just rest for ten minutes and then maybe I'll feel better.' I started resting and I haven't stopped.

At first I just had absolutely devastating exhaustion. I only felt human if I was lying flat and had been for several hours. Doing almost anything was completely exhausting, particularly anything to do with people. I couldn't follow a normal conversation. I was still reading at that stage because my eyes weren't too bad then. I read thrillers and things like that that didn't involve any concentration.

I was working for an organisation called British Refugee Council providing a service to homeless refugees. I was also the shop steward of the trade union there. It was the winter of the miner's strike and it had been an incredibly busy winter and I had really worked hard. It was a very busy, active way of life with a lot of rushing about. I have always been a very energetic person – much more than all of my friends. Everyone always asked how on earth did I have so much energy. But that year I pretty much keeled over.

I was in such a state of exhaustion, literally just dragging myself around, that I went home to my Mum's to rest. The weather was quite nice so I just lay around in the sun and just enjoyed the fact that I had the chance to really rest.

It was three or four weeks before I tried going back to work again. The first day I tried to go back I got about halfway on the Tube and I knew it was really a mistake. I was wondering if I was going to make it to the office I felt so awful. I did make it to work and one of my friends asked how I felt and I said it was like I'd been hit round the head with a sledge hammer. I was completely confused and disorientated and I was still exhausted.

After four weeks of struggling to and from work I tried working part-time in the mornings only. But it was hopeless. It was an incredibly busy office and wasn't really the right place to try. People assumed that I was energetic and back to my old self and I couldn't cope with that.

I was worried I might have glandular fever so I asked my doctor if I could be tested. The test came back negative but it did show that I had had some sort of virus. I think that evidence of viral infection was one of the reasons I got such an early diagnosis of ME.

In July 1985 I was actually diagnosed as having ME by a doctor at Coppett's Wood Hospital where I had been referred by my GP. I had begun to think I might have multiple sclerosis because I had a lot of eye symptoms including double vision, so in a way I was quite relieved when I was told it was ME.

I remember being told it might be ME very vividly. The doctor said I might be ill for two years and that I might never get back my full energy. I was incredibly relieved not to have MS. I saw this as a challenge that if anyone could get better, then it was me. I didn't feel particularly depressed by the diagnosis but I couldn't believe it was going to take two years to recover. That was an inconceivable length of time to be ill. I'd been thinking in terms of 'Will I be better by Monday?'

After that I decided to give up work and find something different to do. The main thing I felt at that stage was that this must be some kind of burnout. I'd been over-active for a long time and it was obviously crazy to carry on doing the same job. I felt that if I set up my life differently and did something less stressful then things would work out.

I applied to do a computing course at London Polytechnic. So I finished work at the end of August 1985 and had some time off before my course started in October.

I looked on this as a sort of rest period when I would get better. I thought it was all psychological that once I'd got myself away from work and onto the course everything would be fine.

It was quite a shock when I started on the course. I thought that I would be better having had the summer off and then I found that I was absolutely no way better. It was a real struggle. My eyes were excruciatingly painful and looking at a computer screen was just a crazy thing to do. It hurt every time I looked at it.

About November time it was beginning to sink home that this was a physical illness. My body had undergone very major changes and it was not the superficial thing I thought it was.

When I'd been ill for six months I gave a Get Well Party. It was really to try and get the people who were closest to me to understand that I needed help. I needed them to be fighting for me to get well so that I could rest and it worked. All my friends came round and we sat in the dark, which is how I had to be most of the time because of my eyes, and I told them about ME.

After that I decided to regulate much more the amount of work I did. I decided I wouldn't work every spare minute of the day but I would only work three or four hours a day. Outside of those hours I would sleep or rest. That began to help a lot because I stopped doing a lot of things that were actually making me ill.

Until then I'd tried to carry on as normal. For instance, I'd gone on holiday with my brother and two other friends to the Lake District. It was meant to be a lovely holiday seeing the countryside. But the others got out and went for great long walks while I just sat in the car at the bottom of the hill feeling really frustrated. So I gave up seeing friends and being with people unless it was going to be relaxing and I was going to enjoy seeing them and still feel well at the end of it. I just felt that I couldn't be with people who were going to be a drain on me. I couldn't cope with hearing other people's problems.

I contacted the ME Association and asked if they knew anyone who had got well after ME and they said they didn't. I went to a few support group meetings but I found them a real strain. I'd spend a couple of hours listening and trying to be helpful to people who were feeling very desperate about having ME which was exactly the kind of thing that everywhere else in my life I was avoiding.

By the spring of 1986 I was starting to feel better. I was

starting to feel just tired rather than absolutely exhausted. It was more a physical tiredness not the kind of overwhelming exhaustion that if I climbed another step or moved another muscle I would be wiped out.

It was all right if I could do things in a relaxed, unhurried state of mind. But anything that made me tense, or if I had to concentrate very hard, would make me ill. I had days when I would feel almost fine and then I'd have a relapse and would have to slow down. I had to learn to take notice when I was beginning to rush and not get caught up in that speediness.

I tried some alternative therapies as well. For about six months, acupuncture seemed to help a great deal with my eyes. I had weekly sessions and occasionally the acupuncturist would give me a homeopathic remedy. When I first went to her she told me I would be cured in six months but by the end of that time she told me that was more or less all she could do for me. I was quite a bit better but I think she was baffled that I hadn't got better than I had. Obviously she didn't admit to that.

Over the summer of 1986 I think I really began to feel better. The course finished and I think in some ways it was the course that kept me ill. Although I was only doing a few hours a day it really was quite hard work. I was growing to understand what I had to do to get well again. I had to be more ruthless in what activities I could and couldn't do. I had to be more open about being ill; I stopped looking after other people and being worried about them. It was the complete opposite to what I'd been before. I was much more ruthless and selfish and decided that getting well mattered more than anything else and I'm going to get well what ever happens.

I think people with ME seem to be very energetic and very responsive to everything around them but they're not very good at looking after themselves. I think ME is a bit like your body's been driven on high patterns of energy for years and years and then it goes on strike and refuses to do anything else until you negotiate new terms and conditions. That's what it was like for me. I've made big changes in my attitude to myself. I'm more important than I used to think I was.

An important stage for me was coming to terms with

anxieties. I had to stop avoiding things that were frightening. Like changing jobs and splitting up with the boyfriend I had been living with. Right now I'm at the stage where I'm persuading my body to break the habit of putting up with these symptoms. I know I'm well and I've got various techniques of reminding myself that I don't have to feel like this. Then a few hours later I usually feel better.

Today I'm much better than I was but I'm not completely cured. I still have double vision almost all the time. I feel slightly dazed and I used to be a very clear-headed sort of person. I used to be very efficient and could remember lots of things. Now I have to write everything down. But I'm sure these things will clear up eventually.

17 Conclusion

ME is still one of the great medical mysteries. The only thing we can say with certainty is that there is, as yet, no cure, and without doubt ME is one of the most difficult of illnesses to live with.

For years sufferers have had to battle for the recognition that their illness is organic. The controversy over the cause of ME has done little to help sufferers who have been labelled as malingerers, hypochondriacs or just afraid of life, and until there is definite proof of a cause the controversy will rage on.

Whilst doing the research for this book the one thing that has amazed us is how little is really known about ME. Why do people with ME feel constantly fatigued? Why are their muscles weak? Why are their sleep patterns disrupted? Why are they so often hypoglycaemic? Why are they so prone to allergies and Candida? And there are many more Whys! What bothers us is that no one is doing this research. Just a handful of doctors are searching for the cause of the illness but no one is looking at the metabolism of ME patients to find out why they suffer such an array of symptoms.

Until a serious, and properly funded, research programme is undertaken we will be no nearer answering any of those questions than we are now. So we come back to the central theme of this book, which is that patients must help themselves.

It is clear that there is very little doctors can do to cure ME. They may be able to relieve symptoms but they cannot offer anything approaching a cure. So patients have got to take things into their own hands.

Most of us are so used to turning up in the doctor's surgery and walking out with a prescription for every ill. ME is not like that. There is no magic bullet and, at this stage, patients would be foolish to expect one. If you have been used to relying on your doctor for the answers to all your health problems you will probably have your illusions shattered. Doctors do not have all the answers and that is particularly so with ME.

As Dr Albert Schweitzer said: 'Each patient carries his own

doctor inside him. They come to us not knowing the truth. We are at our best when we give the doctor who resides within each patient a chance to go to work.'

Of all the sufferers we spoke to who have recovered from ME, the one thing that comes through is that they have all taken responsibility for their health before they could begin to think about recovery.

As Hilary McLennan says, 'A lot of people are desperately looking for a miracle cure – they rush around from consultant to consultant looking for an instant remedy. It's better to look within yourself. Once you've accepted that doctors have not got the answer, that no one has the answer, you realise that you have to handle it yourself. That was the beginning of being able to recover for me.'

The first thing that every ME sufferer should do is find out all they can about their illness. Reading this book will be a start. Now you should join the ME Association or the ME Action Campaign who will keep you informed of the latest developments in research. The ME Association holds regular meetings and an annual conference for doctors and patients to keep them up to date on ME research.

Developing a positive attitude to life may sound flippant to some but it really is the only way you can even start to come to terms with ME. If you allow yourself to get bogged down in the depression that so often accompanies the illness you will never climb back to full health again.

Probably the most important thing is for ME sufferers to tune into themselves and learn to recognise what their bodies are telling them. You have to learn to stop exercising before you are reduced to a state of complete exhaustion. You have to learn to avoid hypoglycaemia. You have to find out which situations will leave you feeling weak and tired – whether it is a dinner party or walking to the shops and standing in a queue at the supermarket.

Many sufferers find it very helpful to keep a diary of their illness. This is time consuming but it serves as a useful record of symptoms, drugs taken and things achieved, and can be invaluable in linking activities and the onset of symptoms.

Above all, you have to listen to what your mind and body are telling you. One of the things that comes through most clearly in any study of ME is that mind and body cannot be separated.

Appendix A

Medical Studies
It has often been said by people who cannot bring themselves to believe in food allergies that there have been no proper trials to establish their existence. In fact there have been several and all reported in major medical magazines. Six of the most important are listed below.

1. 'Food Allergy, Fact or Fiction' – Finn R. and Cohen H. *The Lancet* 25 February 1978.

A double-blind trial of a number of patients with multiple symptoms including tachycardias. Specific food intolerances confirmed by double-blind reintroduction of food by masked and coded syringes and stomach tubes.

2. 'A Critical Study of Clinical Ecology' – R. Finn and I. Battock *The Practitioner* October 1985.

Thirteen of nineteen patients (68 per cent) with hitherto untreatable disease improved on an environmental programme including desensitising injections and dietary manipulation.

3. 'Food Intolerance a Major Factor in the Pathogenesis of the Irritable Bowel Syndrome' – Hunter et al. *The Lancet* November 1982.

Specific foods were found to provoke symptoms of irritable bowel syndrome in 14 of 21 patients. In six patients who were challenged double-blind the food intolerance was confirmed.

4. 'Food Allergies and Migraine' – Ellen C. Grant, *The Lancet* 5 May 1979.

60 patients completed elimination diets. 85 per cent of patients became headache-free.

5. 'Is Migraine Food Allergy?' – J. Soothill et al, *The Lancet* October 1983.

93 per cent of 88 children with severe frequent migraine recovered on oligo-antigenic diets. The causative foods were identified by sequential reintroduction and the role of the foods provoking migraine was established by double-blind controlled trial in 40 of the children.

6. 'Migraine is a Food Allergic Disease' – J. Brostoff et al, *The Lancet* 29 September 1984, 719–721.

Recommended Reading

Books on Allergies
1. Randolph T. & Moss R. – *Allergies – The Hidden Enemy* (Thorsons Publishers, England)
2. Lawrence Dickey (ed.) – *Clinical Ecology* (Charles C. Thomas Publishers, USA)
3. Mackarness, Richard – *Not All in the Mind* (Pan Books, England)
4. Mackarness, Richard – *Chemical Victims* (Pan Books, England)
5. Eagle, Robert – *Eating And Allergy* (Thorsons Publishers, England)
6. Mansfield, John – *The Migraine Revolution* (Thorsons Publishers, England)
7. Mumby, Keith – *Food Allergy Plan* (Unwin-Hyman Ltd, England)
8. Mumby, Keith – *Allergies: What Everyone Should Know* (Unwin-Hyman Ltd, England)
9. Brostoff J. and Challacombe D.M. (eds.) – *Food Allergy and Intolerance* (Baillière, Tindall, England)
10. Mansfield, Peter and Monro, Jean – *Chemical Children* (Century Hutchinson Ltd, England)
11. Mumby, Keith – *The Allergy Handbook* (Thorsons Publishers, England. October 1988, the most up to date of all)

Appendix A

Books and Articles on ME

1. Mayne, Michael – *A Year Lost and Found* (Darton, Longman & Todd, England)
2. Ramsay, Melvin – *Post-Viral Fatigue Syndrome* (The ME Association, England)
3. Ho-Yen, Darrel – *Better Recovery from Viral Illnesses* (Dodona Books, The Old Schoolhouse, Inverness, Scotland)
4. *Meeting Place*, the journal of ANZMES, the Australia and New Zealand ME Society, PO Box 35/429, Browns Bay, Auckland 10, New Zealand.
5. Steincamp J. and Catley C. – *Overload: Beating ME* (Whatamongo Bay, Queen Charlotte Sound, New Zealand. Very up-to-date and particularly recommended)
6. Acheson, E.D. – 'Encephalomyelitis associated with poliomyelitis virus' *(The Lancet* 2, 1044–1048)
7. Acheson, E.D. – 'The clinical syndrome variously called Benign Myalgic Encephalomyelitis, Iceland Disease and Epidemic Neuromyasthenia' *(American Journal of Medicine*, 26, 569–595)
8. Behan, P.O., Behan W.M.H. & Bell E.J. – 'The post-viral fatigue syndrome: an analysis of the findings in 50 cases' *(Journal of Infection*, 10, 211–222)
9. Keighley, B.D. & Bell E.J. – 'Sporadic myalgic encephalomyelitis in a rural practice' *(Journal of General Practitioners*, 33, 339–341)
10. McEvedy, C.P. & Beard, A.W. – 'Royal Free epidemic of 1955: a reconsideration' *(British Medical Journal*, 1, 7–11)
11. McEvedy, C.P. & Beard, A.W. – 'Concept of Benign Myalgic Encephalomyelitis' *(British Medical Journal*, 1, 11–15)
12. McEvedy, C.P. Griffith A. & Hall T. – 'Two School Epidemics' *(British Medical Journal*, 2, 1300)
13. Moss, P.D. & McEvedy, C.P. – 'An epidemic of overbreathing among schoolgirls' *(British Medical Journal*, 2, 1295–1300)
14. Ramsay, A.M. – 'Encephalomyelitis simulating poliomyelitis and hysteria' *(The Lancet*, 2, 1196–1200)
15. Ramsay, A.M. & O'Sullivan E. – 'Encephalomyelitis simulating poliomyelitis' *(The Lancet*, 1, 761–766)
16. Southern, P. & Oldstone, M.B.A. – 'Medical consequences of persistent viral infections' *(New England Journal of Medicine*, 314, 359–367)

17. Straus, S.E., Tosato, G. & Armstrong, G. – 'Persisting illness and fatigue in adults with evidence of Epstein-Barr virus infection' *(Annals of Internal Medicine,* 102, 7–18)
18. David, A., Wessely S., Pelosi, A. – 'Post Viral Fatigue Syndrome – Time for a New Approach' *(British Medical Journal,* 1988, 1, 696–698)
19. Yousef, G. et al. – 'Chronic Enterovirus infection in Patients with Post Viral Fatigue Syndrome' *(The Lancet* 1988: 1, 146-149)

Books on Candida

1. Trowbridge, John & Walker, M. – *The Yeast Syndrome* (Bantam Books, USA)
2. Crook, William – *The Yeast Connection* (Random House, England)
3. Chaitow, Leon – *Candida Albicans: Is Yeast Your Problem?* (Thorsons Publishers, England)
4. Truss, Orian – *The Missing Diagnosis* (Birmingham, Alabama, USA)
5. Kingsley, Patrick – *Conquering Cystitis* (Ebury Press, England)

Books on Nutrition

1. Kenton, L. & S. – *Raw Energy* (Century Hutchinson, England)
2. Davies, S. & Stewart, A. – *Nutritional Medicine* (Pan Books, England)
3. Holford, Patrick – *The Family Nutrition Workbook* (Thorsons Publishers, England)
4. Holford, Patrick – *Vitamin Vitality* (Collins Publishers, England)
5. Pauling, Linus – *How to Live Longer and Feel Better* (Freeman Publishers, USA)
6. Stone, Irving – *Vitamin C Against Disease* (Grosset & Dunlap, USA)
7. Graham, Judy – *Evening Primrose Oil* (Thorsons Publishers, England)

General

1. Phillpot W. and Kalita D. – *Brain Allergies: The Psycho-Nutrient Connection* (Keats Publishers, USA)

2. Sheinkin & Schackter – *Food, Mind and Mood* (Warner Books, USA)
3. Selye, Hans – *Stress and Life* (McGraw-Hill, USA)
4. Siegel, B. – *Love, Medicine and Miracles* (Century Hutchinson, England)
5. Lidell, L. – *The Book of Massage: The Complete Step by Step Guide to Eastern and Western Techniques* (Ebury Press, England).

Appendix B

Useful addresses for ME Sufferers

Action Against Allergy, 43 The Downs, London SW20

British Acupuncture Association and Register, 22 Hockley Road, Rayleigh, Essex SS6 8EB

British Homeopathic Association, 27a Devonshire Street, London W1N 1RJ

British Medical Acupuncture Association, 67–69 Chancery Lane, London WC2A 1AE

British Society of Medical and Dental Hypnosis, 42 Links Road, Ashtead, Surrey KT21 2HJ

Citizens Rights Office, Child Poverty Action Group, 1 Machlis Street, London WC2B 5MH

The Disability Alliance, 25 Denmark Street, London WC2H 5NH

General Council and Register of Consultant Herbalists Ltd, Marlborough House, Swanpool, Falmouth, Cornwall TR11 4HW

Institute for Complementary Medicine, 21 Portland Place, London W1N 3AE

ME Action Campaign, PO Box 1126, London W3 0RY

ME Association, PO Box 8, Stanford-le-Hope, Essex SS17 8BX

Social Security advice from your local Social Security Office (look in the phone book under Social Security or Health and Social Security). A free telephone information service is available to answer general enquiries, remember the people answering the phone will not have your file to hand so will only be able to give general information. Ring 0800–666555.

Society for Environmental Therapy, 3 Atherton Road, Ipswich, Suffolk

ANZMES, the Australia and New Zealand ME Society, PO Box 35/429, Browns Bay, Auckland 10, New Zealand

British Society for Nutritional Medicine, PO Box 3AP, London W1A 3AP.

British Society of Allergy and Environmental Medicine, 34 Brighton Road, Banstead, Surrey SM17 1BS

Lamberts Dietary Products, 1 Lamberts Road, Tunbridge Wells, TN2 3EQ, supplier of hypoallergenic vitamins and minerals.

Australia

ME Society, PO Box 645, Mona Vale, NSW 2103

ME Society, PO Box 7, Moonee Ponds, VIC 3039

Allergy Association, Australia – New South Wales, PO Box 74, Sylvania, Southgate, NSW 2224

Australian Society for Environmental Medicine: Suite 4, Collins Street, Melbourne, Vic 3000

New Zealand

Christchurch ME Support Group, Po Box 143, Christchurch

Auckland Allergy Awareness Association Inc, Box 12–701, Penrose

Wellington Hyperactivity & Allergy Association, 93 Waipapa Road, Wellington 3

Foundation for the Healing Arts, PO Box 4529, Christchurch

USA

National Chronic Fatigue Association Inc, PO Box 230108, Portland, Oregon

Appendix B

Human Environmental Medicine Inc, 6386 Alvorado Court, San Diego, CA92120

The CFIDS Association, PO Box 220398, Charlotte, North Carolina 28222

Index

Index

177